Growth Monitoring and Promotion in Young Children

Growth Monitoring and Promotion in Young Children

Guidelines for the Selection of Methods and Training Techniques

DERRICK B. JELLIFFE, M.D.
Professor of Public Health and Pediatrics
Chairman, IUNS Working Group II/1

E. F. PATRICE JELLIFFE, M.P.H.
Lecturer, Population and Family Health Division
Chairperson, IUNS Committee IV/6

School of Public Health,
University of California,
Los Angeles

New York   Oxford
OXFORD UNIVERSITY PRESS
1990

The authors gratefully acknowledge the assistance of the IUNS, UNICEF, and WHO in the preparation of this book.

Oxford University Press

Oxford   New York   Toronto
Delhi   Bombay   Calcutta   Madras   Karachi
Petaling Jaya   Singapore   Hong Kong   Tokyo
Nairobi   Dar es Salaam   Cape Town
Melbourne   Auckland

and associated companies in
Berlin   Ibadan

Library of Congress Cataloging-in-Publication Data
Jelliffe, Derrick Brian.
Growth monitoring and promotion in young children : guidelines
for the selection of methods and training techniques /
Derrick B. Jelliffe and E. F. Patrice Jelliffe.
p. cm.   Includes bibliographical references.
ISBN 0-19-505623-X
1. Children—Growth—Tables.   2. Children—Growth—Forecasting.
3. Children—Developing countries—Growth.
I. Jelliffe, E. F. Patrice.   II. Title.
RJ131.J38   1990
612.6′54—dc20   89-23085   CIP

1 2 3 4 5 6 7 8 9
Printed in the United States of America
on acid-free paper

Preface

The invisible slowing down of normal growth happens long before a child becomes malnourished. Regular monthly weighing
and the use of a child growth chart can make visible this faltering
growth and so provide an early warning to mothers and health
workers.

James Grant (1985)

The concept of growth monitoring [is] an outgrowth of nutritional
status assessment, but aimed at intervention before malnutrition
becomes evident.

Hendrata and Rohde (1988)

Growth monitoring: intermediate technology or expensive luxury?

Editorial: *Lancet* (1985)

The apparently self-evident value of growth monitoring in early childhood has
been questioned in recent years. It has become recognized that this is by no
means always a simple, economical procedure that has an automatic effect on
a child's nutritional status. Some of the current confusion is indicated by the
preceding quotations. Relevant issues include the affordability of large numbers
of low-cost scales for national programs, cultural difficulties with illiterate
community health workers and mothers in using and understanding growth charts,
and even differences in the definition of "monitoring."

This book addresses these and other controversial issues. The text is based
in part on an IUNS (International Union of Nutritional Sciences) meeting, sup-
ported by UNICEF and WHO. Participants are acknowledged later. It also incorporates a review of recent literature, together with correspondence and advice from colleagues in different parts of the world.

This book is intended to complement several excellent publications by UNI-
CEF (Hendrata, 1988), WHO (1978b), the American Public Health Association
(Griffiths, 1981a), and a special supplement of the *Indian Journal of Pediatrics*
(1988). Together, these could comprise a small growth monitoring reference
library, as suggested in the bibliography, to assist the difficult choices that need
to be made in selecting methods for differing circumstances.

*It is not intended as a universal training manual or guide to one guaranteed
method of growth monitoring of worldwide usefulness and easy application. In*

fact, none exists. Instead, the book will indicate the need for selection from a range of options and alternatives, so that appropriate methods can be selected that fit within national economic constraints. A range of systems exists from what has been termed "ideal" in this book (pp. 60, 65), to less complex compromise systems, which are feasible locally and can still be helpful, to situations where any form of growth monitoring may be impossible with current resources and circumstances.

Inevitably, this poses more problems of choice than if one universal system could be advocated, as was at one time believed. Such discussion exposes some areas of disagreement as well as the need for field trials of methods and instruments in different circumstances, using several more innovative but as yet inadequately tested procedures. As will be discussed, objectives and uses of growth monitoring programs can vary. Nowhere is growth monitoring a precise analytical procedure. It is intended as a general diagnostic guide to action and, hopefully, an educational stimulus for parents and health workers (Gopalan, 1987).

Three seemingly obvious themes for effective growth monitoring and promotion that have recently been disputed and discussed are emphasized in this book. These have been summarized recently by Pradilla (1987):

- Growth monitoring *is* a useful tool.
- Methods and specific tools for carrying out monitoring have to be designed according to the people using them.
- A critical issue is how to respond to decreased velocity of growth. Here again, what can be done in every location is the basic constraint. The principle is to do something useful, if monitoring is to have any use.

Recently emphasized difficulties in growth monitoring may sometimes be related to the fact that the objectives of some programs need to be rethought and their organization modified, as made necessary by local limitations and constraints. These include the methods used in training or other seemingly straightforward procedures. For example, Hendrata and Rohde (1988) have described "ten commonly encountered pitfalls" that are often responsible for failure (p. 7).

This book explores these and other pitfalls and indicates improvements or alternative methods capable of detecting early growth failure and promoting optimal growth. Both elements—monitoring and promotion—are needed and depend for success on the orientation and modification of the program toward *realistic training of staff, effective communication with and motivation of mothers, and feasible action,* based as much as possible on community involvement.

Los Angeles   D.B.J.
October 1989   E.F.P.J.

Contents

I

BACKGROUND

1

Growth Monitoring for Health Promotion

Much like a thermometer that can provide a health worker a reading about fever in a sick child, so can a growth chart tell a health worker vital information about the nutritional well being of an individual child.

Jean Baker (1986)

The original meaning of "monitoring" is to remind or give warning. Growth monitoring consists of measuring, recording, and interpreting an individual's growth over a sufficient period of time. It is an important part of health supervision and promotion, especially at those stages of life when rapid growth normally occurs. These include pregnancy, the neonatal period, infancy, and childhood. Worldwide, however, growth monitoring is particularly employed with young children in the first 5 years of life—during infancy and the so-called preschool period. In addition, practical methods of maternal-fetal monitoring are being investigated and increasingly used in many parts of the world.

Growth monitoring in early childhood is intended as a tool to (1) promote and sustain good health and growth in this vulnerable age group and (2) detect early growth failure due to an inadequate diet, infections, social influences or, very often, a combination of these factors. It has become an essential part of "child survival programs" in primary health care services. It can be an indicator not only of dietary inadequacy, but also of the effects of diarrhea (especially if incorrectly treated) and of infections potentially preventable by immunization.

There sometimes seems to be a lack of understanding of the difference between two objectives—*growth monitoring versus growth promotion* (Hendrata & Rohde, 1988). Growth monitoring usually refers to the early detection of malnutrition or ill health by serial measurements during the period of childhood when this occurs most commonly, often the second year of life (Morley, 1968). Growth promotion focuses on maintaining and promoting normal growth from birth. These two overlapping objectives need different emphases in practice and training in view of the different age groups involved.

Whenever possible, both objectives—often abbreviated to GM/P—need to be included, but the promotion of optimal growth from birth or early infancy is the ideal as a truly preventive measure. However, as Ghosh (1977) commented in India, "Children have [usually] been weighed perfunctorily to assess levels and extent of malnutrition rather than to determine growth as one of the most important indications of health."

Whatever their main purpose, periodic weighing or other measurements are only methods of estimating growth. They do not reveal the causes of abnormalities. They are a useless and sterile exercise unless followed by appropriate interpretation and action (Nabarro and Chinnock, 1988). Both the detection of the main causes and clearly defined, locally feasible actions need to be essential parts of whatever process is possible in local circumstances. Alternatives are outlined later (Chapter 4).

Growth monitoring and nutrition assessment have been confused in the past because anthropometry is used in both (Jelliffe & Jelliffe, 1989). Indeed, there can be an overlap. Anthropometric measurements are mainstays of surveys, screening, and surveillance for nutrition status. Analysis of records of growth monitoring charts can form part of the nutrition assessment of communities (Appendix A). However, growth monitoring is "more than the collection of data" (Griffiths, 1988).

Growth can be monitored by measuring body dimensions. *Relevant measurements* (whether weight, height, or arm circumference), *types of equipment available* (or needed), the *frequency of assessment,* and the *interpretation of findings* will vary for different ages and the purposes of different programs. Very frequent measurements are best for monitoring in the early weeks or months of life when growth should be rapid, yet cultural and logistical problems may make this difficult (Chapter 3).

Some aspects of growth monitoring have been incorporated into "nutritional support services," including parenteral nutrition, in sophisticated hospitals and in the management of endocrine and metabolic disorders. There has been much recent work on monitoring fetal growth with modern technology, such as ultrasound, and with uncomplicated "appropriate technology" used by community health workers in less technically developed countries, such as recording maternal weight gain and increase in fundal height in pregnancy. Various forms of growth monitoring now comprise an essential part of maternal and child care and health supervision in the pediatric and obstetrical services of high-technology hospitals and research centers as well as in the community work of primary health care services everywhere, especially in less technically developed countries.

It has long been appreciated that growth is a characteristic of healthy childhood and that its measurement is "one of the most important tools of the pediatrician's trade" (Grant, 1987). Nevertheless, *practical details* of how to carry out measurements and how to detect early growth failure often are not given much emphasis in medical education, despite the availability in recent decades of elaborate centile graphs of weight, height, and head circumference for boys and girls. Such tasks are commonly regarded as technically simple and *in practice* are not included in the training of medical students and interns.

More often than not, health professionals in many countries have little or no idea to what the various locally used lines on weight graphs refer. As an example of this lack of clarity, "failure to thrive" is vaguely defined in the eleventh edition of Nelson's classic *Textbook of Pediatrics* as "failure to gain weight or to grow at the expected rate" (Barbero & McKay, 1979). Adequacy of growth has often been judged by comparison with average figures of weight gain per week or month or a longer period, which can vary considerably between children and during different times in their lives, since growth in normal, healthy children is not a smooth, uninterrupted process.

By contrast, specialists concerned with detailed aspects of growth, such as auxologists (who study growth of all body components) and endocrinologists, have devised refined charts for measuring incremental growth velocity (Roche & Hines, 1980) and have developed precise but expensive scientific instruments for making a wide range of body measurements. These do not have wide applications outside advanced medical centers.

Because protein-energy malnutrition is so common and serious in young children in less technically developed countries, Morley (1968) introduced simplified "Road-to-Health" weight charts, employing the calendar system, some 30 years ago. These were intended mainly for use in child health services in Third World countries. They were meant to be scientifically based but were never intended principally for nutritional diagnosis. Their main purpose was to help the health worker and the consumer (i.e., the mother) to understand the importance of sustaining growth and to recognize failure to gain weight, shown visibly on the graph, as an indication of ill health needing appropriate investigation and action.

With support from WHO, UNICEF, and many nongovernmental organizations (NGO), relatively simplified weight charts have now come into use in many countries. Growth monitoring almost always forms a major activity in what have come to be termed primary health care "Child Survival and Development Strategies" or "Child Survival Programmes" (Grant, 1985, 1987). As part of this movement, many modifications have been made in weight charts in different countries, and a very variable amount of other information has been included on the card, called a home-based child record (HBCR) or child health passport (Sinha, 1986), which is retained by the mother.

Currently, it has been estimated that 200 to 300 different cards are in use in more than 80 countries. Some are quite similar to the original Morley Road-to-Health chart, subsequently revised by WHO (1978). Some show marked differences, such as several additional lines indicating different levels of underweight and, in a few instances, levels of overweight as well.

In the past 2 or 3 years, the value of growth charts has been questioned for a variety of reasons by different workers. Particular mention may be made of valuably constructive reviews of growth monitoring by Gopalan and Chatterjee (1986) and Nabarro and Chinnock (1988).

Such critical reviews have emphasized *poor training* (and consequent inaccuracy both in measuring and recording), the *relatively high cost of equipment,* the *large numbers of children* likedly to be involved, the *time spent* (compared with other activities), the frequent unavailability of worthwhile, reachable *support services* for supervision and referral, and the *difficulties with the interpretation of growth charts for action* by community health workers or supervisors.

Some programs have devoted the most attention to *coverage*—that is, the number of children measured. More (but not enough) have emphasized the detailed mechanics of monitoring (usually weighing and charting), though often without sufficient simplification and practical instruction. The least attention has been given to interpreting findings, indicating appropriate action(s), and developing methods for the real, practical involvement of mothers in the whole process.

These points can be best understood when considering the five main tasks that need to be undertaken in growth monitoring by the responsible workers in "health teams" in the community (including mothers)—*motivating* mothers to bring their children and become involved in the whole process, *measuring* weight accurately, *recording* on often culturally unfamiliar graphs, *interpreting* the child's condition from the growth and other evidence, and *taking appropriate action* in the local circumstances (Fig. 1-1). Details concerning the improvement and variation of these five stages are given later.

In primary health care services for children, different tasks in this five-stage sequence may be carried out by physicians or nurses. However, they are usually the responsibility of community health workers, who tend to be minimally paid, to have limited education, and to be occupied with several other duties (Williams et al., 1986). Health care workers usually must motivate mothers to attend the clinic and become involved in growth monitoring and must advise them on various matters, including feeding and prevention and management of infections. In many places, some degree of practical involvement of mothers has been obtained, but it is often lacking and the whole process then becomes a mysterious ritual (McGuire & Austin, 1987). In a few areas, however, major activities have been undertaken by the mothers themselves (Rohde et al., 1978; Arole, 1988). In some other circumstances, older school children have participated in child-to-child programs (Aarons & Hawes, 1979) in weighing their younger siblings.

The site for growth monitoring also varies. Often it is a community health worker clinic, village center, or neighborhood collecting center; or monitoring

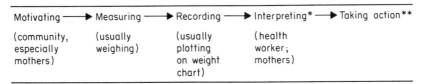

Motivating ⟶	Measuring ⟶	Recording ⟶	Interpreting* ⟶	Taking action**
(community, especially mothers)	(usually weighing)	(usually plotting on weight chart)	(health worker; mothers)	

* Growth and other information described later (Chapter 4).
** Motivation, understanding, and combined action by health worker, mother, and family.

Figure 1-1   Sequence of five activities or tasks in growth monitoring.

Table 1-1 Ten common pitfalls of growth monitoring and promotion (GM/P)

1. The curative approach to nutritional problems.
2. Focus on the wrong age.
3. Nutritional status rather than growth is emphasized.
4. Lack of feedback.
5. No individualized advice or interaction.
6. Belief that GM/P is simple and therefore must be easy.
7. GM/P is seen and conducted as an isolated activity related to nutrition.
8. Lack of community involvement.
9. Food takes over the central stage.
10. False expectations abound, as to value of monitoring as an effective intervention without subsequent action.

Modified from Hendrata & Rohde, 1988.

is carried out in the course of home visiting. Alternatively, less frequent weighing sessions may be held at intervals of several months at selected rallying points.

Travel to a clinic or village center can be time consuming for mothers. Home visiting encroaches on the limited time available to community health workers, but it does permit them to observe the home circumstances and to note potential risk factors. Thus, it can help stimulate those at greatest risk and remind defaulters of the need to attend clinics or centers.

Weighings at collecting points at widely spaced intervals of several months may be all that is possible in some circumstances. This can only serve as a rough measure for individual growth monitoring and is of even less value in growth promotion. However, it does provide a method of diagnosing the situation in a community and an imperfect, intermittent screening process to detect malnourished children.

The variety of sites for growth monitoring bears emphasizing, as it is often assumed that the activity is only carried out at a static, orthodox clinic. This is not so. Indeed, the expression ''child clinic'' can itself cover a wide range of different settings, from hospital outpatient clinics to health centers to informal village gatherings organized by a resident or visiting community health worker.

Problems and difficulties can occur at all of the stages mentioned (Fig. 1-1), with the possibility of cumulative errors and misunderstandings resulting. As emphasized by WHO (1978b) and UNICEF (1988), it has become timely to review the value, limitations, and pitfalls (Table 1-1) of current growth monitoring systems, consider alternative ways of monitoring growth, and adapt and improve existing practices when indicated and practicable.

This book forms part of such a reappraisal, with special reference to the selection of alternative methods of growth monitoring and improving training, particularly involving mothers. Interpretation and practical action, as well as innovative technical procedures, are also emphasized.

Selection of economical methods of measurement, recording, and training are key concerns everywhere. This tends to become more so when the coverage by primary health care services increases rapidly with limited resources, as has happened in some countries in recent years. Details of any effective training program also have to depend on a realistic understanding of the range of methods and tools actually or potentially available and feasible in very variable circumstances in different areas of the world.

2

Tools for Growth Monitoring

PRINCIPLES OF SELECTION

In less technically developed regions, growth monitoring will concentrate on vulnerable young children. As noted, major objectives are both to sustain optimal or adequate weight gain and to identify "invisible" malnutrition (Grant, 1987) not obvious to the naked eye (Gopalan, 1987) as early as possible by observing slowing of normal growth. These two objectives have usually been undertaken by serial weighing and recording graphically on whatever chart or record is used locally.

When preliminary screening is all that is practicable, weighing is done at collecting points at intervals of several months, or the arm circumference is measured.

Thus, in some difficult circumstances attempts at growth maintenance may be all that is possible, using arm circumference measurements, which do not alter significantly from 1 to 4 years. This practical, but experimental, alternative is discussed later (Chapter 5).

In rare and especially well-equipped circumstances, height (or length) may be measured as well as weight to assess weight for height serially. This can also differentiate wasted (thin) children from stunted (dwarfed) children (Waterlow et al., 1980).

In all forms of growth monitoring, two items are needed: a *measuring instrument* (usually weighing scales) and a form of *serial record* (usually a weight chart or graph). The selection of these two items depends on many varying factors such as cost, literacy, cultural considerations, educational level of the health workers concerned, ease of use and understandability by workers and mothers, and number of children to be measured. Various alternatives and the advantages of different measuring instruments are discussed elsewhere (Griffiths, 1981; WHO, 1986a; Burns & Rohde, 1988; Jelliffe & Jelliffe, 1989). Some considerations will also be summarized here, since the content and type of training needed obviously has to be related to the equipment used and the method of growth monitoring selected.

MEASURING INSTRUMENTS

Weighing Scales

Weighing scales are most commonly used in growth monitoring; either hanging (suspended) or stand-on scales (floor level or ground scales) are used. Basically, these should be inexpensive, sufficiently accurate, easy to read, easy to transport with a carrying device, and durable enough to have a long life even with rough treatment. Five types of evaluation criteria have been described by Burns and Rohde (1988) (Table 2-1), who also suggested a point system for each feature so that different scales can be compared (Appendix B).

The price is often a major consideration in poor countries where large numbers of scales are needed at first and some replacements thereafter. Two models have been most widely employed: the *Salter circular dial spring scale* (Fig. 2-1a) (measuring up to 25 kg or 60 lb), usually with markings at 100 g (or ¼ lb) and 500 g (or 1 lb) on the dial and, in some countries, a low-cost *local traditional beam-balance scale* (Fig. 2-1b) (as used in Indonesia and the Philippines). The markings and subdivisions on the scale, including those on the dial of the spring scale, should correspond to those on the growth chart. This is especially helpful for a semiliterate community health worker, who may be educationally and culturally unfamiliar both with the decimal system and with reading a circular dial.

Salter scales are often stated to have a 5-year life span, but this obviously depends on the amount of use and the care taken. In some countries, Salter-type scales are manufactured locally, but often with a less certain product and an increased need for testing. Their cost may be lower than that of imported

Table 2-1 Five categories of evaluation criteria for weighing scales

1. The important *criteria in fundamental design* are maintenance, safety, durability, portability, and universality, as well as the ability to tare or reset to zero.

2. The *scale acceptability* questions are based on ease of use for the operator, cultural acceptability for the mother, and comfort for the child.

3. The *potential for scale error* is based on its inherent accuracy, linearity (the ability to measure the the same accuracy over a range of weight), hysteresis (reading accuracy affected by previous load), precision (consistency of a reading), and sensitivity (the least change in a load that can be indicated). In addition, error can be affected by inapparent damage to internal parts or fatigue of the pivotal and essential mechanisms.

4. Analysis of the *potential for operator error* is based on accuracy with regard to simplicity of use and ease of reading, especially parallax (a visual distortion that occurs when the operator gets a different reading depending on the viewing angle).

5. *General criteria* relates to the cost of the scale, its packaging, the type of instructions that accompany it, and the possibility for manufacture in the country of use.

From Burns & Rohde, 1988.

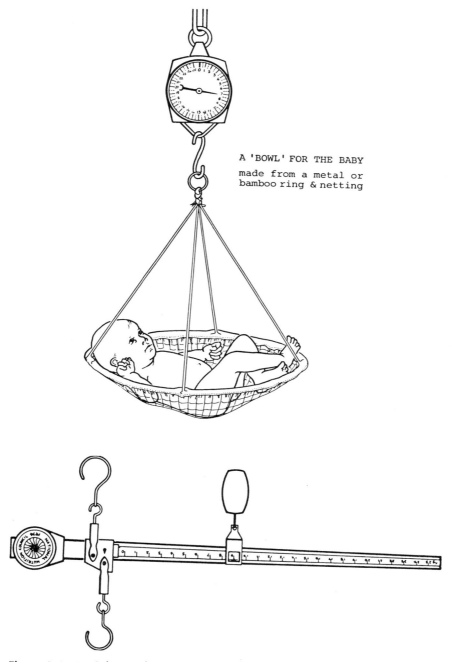

A 'BOWL' FOR THE BABY

made from a metal or
bamboo ring & netting

Figure 2-1 (a) Salter scale (courtesy Professor David Morley). (b) Philippine bar scale (courtesy Nutrition Center of the Philippines).

scales, but this is not necessarily so. Various minor technical modifications have been introduced with regard to the suspension or suspender on which the child is placed during the weighing procedure to minimize anxiety and the oscillation caused by a frightened child (Wilkinson, 1982).

Appropriate test weights are needed to standardize the scales—that is, to check their accuracy after they have been tared, or reset to zero. These can be expensive if known weights from a National Bureau of Standards are used (where such exist). More simply, large plastic containers of known volume can be used and filled with water when required. They are especially valuable if mobile work is entailed. Scales should be tested frequently through the expected range, and certainly before each weighing session.

Efforts have been made to decrease the cost of scales, improve their readability, and simplify plotting on the weight chart. The TALC spring scale, costing about $5 in 1988, allows direct plotting of the weight on the chart with the built-in biro point (Morley, 1986) (Figs. 2-2 and 2-3). A newly developed Sensor International Electronic Scale has recently been developed. It is a solar-powered, direct readout scale with an estimated cost of about $40 for the walk-on model (1988). It is still in an early experimental stage.

These relatively low-cost, easy-to-read innovations may be expected to decrease in price with large-scale production. They are under trial in various parts of the world. Preliminary results with the TALC scale in Sierra Leone and Liberia are promising.

Both scales are intended to make weighing and/or recording easier. If found to be satisfactory, they could greatly modify and simplify training and field work.

Arm Circumference Tapes and Bands

The arm circumference in young children principally reflects stores of calories (subcutaneous fat) and protein (muscle). In healthy children, it does not alter much between 12 and 59 months (Jelliffe & Jelliffe, 1969), and a midpoint (often 16 cm) can be used as a reference level for this age range. However, this reference level may be less appropriate for genetically slim-limbed peoples. The arm circumference reflects the presence of, and recovery from, thinness. Unless obesity develops, it will not increase beyond the reference level.

The upper arm circumference can be measured with a variety of nonstretch tapes. A Zerfas insertion type of tape (Figs. 2-4a and 2-4b) is preferred. It can be read relatively precisely with the least likelihood of overcompression of the arm (Zerfas, 1975).

For *screening* purposes in illiterate communities, colored arm bands have been used. The Shakir tricolor ("traffic lights") tape (Figs. 2-5a and 2-5b) is appropriate for screening in the home (Shakir & Morley, 1974), but not for monitoring at frequent intervals. It is cheap, rapidly replaceable, and easily carried by the community health worker. However, the usual model only differentiates the severe (red) from the apparently normal (green), as there is just

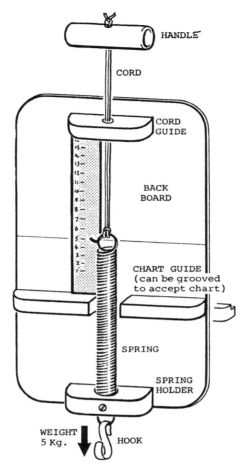

Figure 2-2 TALC scale showing individual parts. A standard Morley weight chart (30 cm × 22 cm) can be slipped into the groove guide to the correct month. The infant's weight can be marked directly on the inserted chart by the biro tip at the top of the spring (courtesy Professor David Morley).

a small yellow band (1 cm) for moderate thinness or underweight. Different colors may have to be used, because colors can have varying significance in different societies. In some cultures, for example, red may be inappropriate as a signal of danger as it implies health.

For greater capacity to detect moderate thinness, Zeitlin et al. (1982) devised a tape to measure thigh circumference. Because the thigh is much larger than the arm, it is easier to detect alterations in measurements. This has not been used in practice.

With illiterate workers in mind, Zeitlin et al. (1982) have tried a four-color arm band, with red, orange, yellow, and white zones indicating varying levels

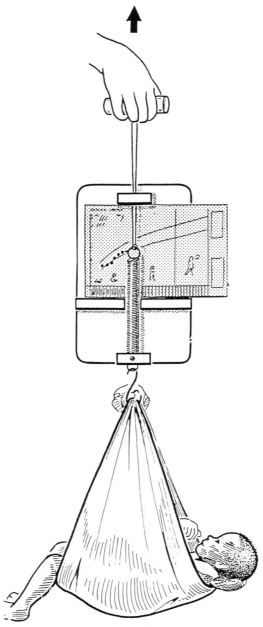

Figure 2-3 TALC scale (courtesy Professor David Morley). A recent version is under trial with a plastic spring or guide.

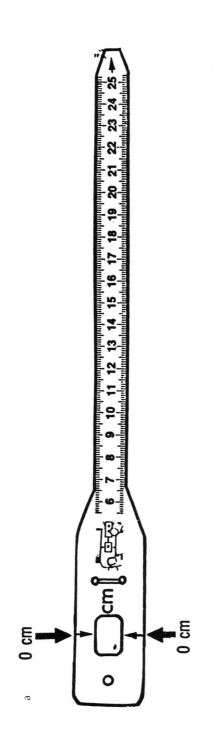

Figure 2-4 Zerfas insertion tapes (courtesy A. Zerfas). (a) Regular Zerfas insertion tape. (b) *Modified tape*, using millimeters and 2-mm intervals, for measuring the arm circumference of young child or pregnant woman, or the fundal height in pregnancy as a rough method of monitoring fetal growth. (Available from TALC, P.O. Box 49, St. Albans, U.K.)

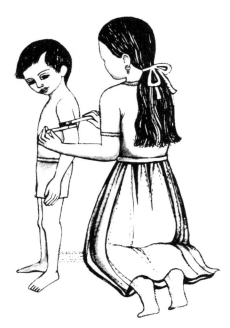

a

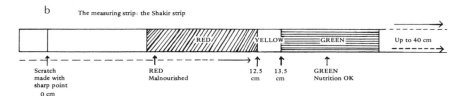

b   The measuring strip: the Shakir strip

Figure 2-5   (a) Shakir arm band (strip or tape) (courtesy Aaron & Hawes, 1979). (b) Shakir tricolor arm circumference tape (detachable) with instructions for use by community health workers in Nepal (green 13.5 to 16 cm, yellow 13.5 to 12.5, red < 12.5.). Tape: right of illustration.

of thinness from severe to normal [suggested measurements: 13.5, 12.5, and 9.5 cm (Zeitlin et al., 1982) or appropriate locally useful levels]. Results can be recorded on a color-coded table.

Other modifications of color-coded arm bands are being tested, possibly with eight zones indicating different levels of thinness and preferably using an insertion type of tape. These will have to be tried out locally to enable the usefulness of serial measurements to be tested as an *approximate* alternative for growth monitoring by repeated weighings.

Results with arm circumference measurements in malnourished children will

कमसेकम दुई वर्ष सम्म बच्चालाई

पाखुराको गोलाईको नापबाट एक देखि पाच वर्ष सम्मको बच्चाहरुको पालन–पोषण बारे सजिलैसंग पत्ता लगाउन सकिन्छ ।

नाप्ने फित्ता प्रयोग गर्ने तरीका

नाप्ने फित्ताको कालो भाग बच्चाको देब्रे पाखुराको कुईनो र कुमको ठीक बीचमा पर्ने गरी बिस्तारै दबाएर राख्नुहोस् । फित्ताले नाप लिंदा बच्चाको हात मोझो र खुकुलोसंग भुण्डिरहेको हुनुपर्छ ।

नाप्ने फित्ताको नाप बुझ्ने तरीका

नाप्ने फित्ताको कालो अंशले त्यही फित्ताको रातो, पहेंलो अथवा हरियो भागमा कुनलाई छोएको छ हेर्नुहोस् ।

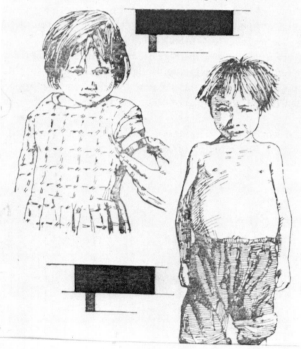

GREEN

YELLOW

RED

स्वस्थ बच्चाको नाप नाप्ने फित्ताको कालो

Figure 2-5b Shakir tricolor arm circumference tape (detachable) with instructions for use by community health workers in Nepal (Green 13.5–16 cm, yellow 13.5–12.5, red < 12.5.) Tape: center of illustration.

not be identical with weight for age (Margo, 1976), but will reflect similar situations. However, as mentioned elsewhere, the arm circumference remains more or less constant in nonobese young children in this age range. After reaching the normal level, it cannot be used for monitoring increase in growth, but it may be used as an approximate measure for *growth maintenance,* as judged by *maintaining* the arm circumference at or above a locally defined level (possibly 15 cm).

Height

It is rarely practical to measure height—or length during the first two years of life—in primary health care settings within less technically developed countries. There is insufficient time and money. Because of the high cost of commercially available equipment, a length/height board has to be constructed locally, and the measurement of a young child requires the combined efforts of three people. Also, little immediately useful information is obtained, as height normally increases slowly and does not decrease with malnutrition. However, serial length/height measurements can be used to detect growth retardation if they are made at long intervals (3 to 6 months).

However, in some circumstances with more resources and a smaller population to be served, length/height measurements have been included. This has been the case in some Caribbean countries (Sinha, 1986) when its purpose was to *graph* the weight for height and to differentiate the stunted from the wasted. This is most unusual.

In other parts of the world, the "Thinness Chart" (Fig. 2-6) has been used to identify children with a low weight for height (Navarro & McNab, 1980).

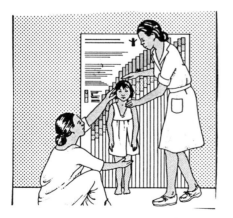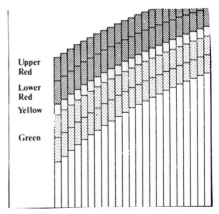

Figure 2-6 Thinness chart (Nabarro & McNab, 1980). Child is weighed and stood in front of approximate weight column. The weight for height is read off according to the color reached by the child's head. Red indicates a low weight for height ("thinness") and green a normal weight for height.

A transportable model has been devised and used in Africa (Campbell et al., 1985) and elsewhere. A floor model of the same chart has been developed to measure the length of young children who are unable to stand, but it does not seem to have been used widely.

The regular Thinness Chart is fixed to the clinic wall. After weighing, the child stands against the chart at the appropriate place for his or her weight, and the weight-for-height category can be read off directly on the chart. It has the advantage of being an age-independent, relatively inexpensive measure that makes it possible to differentiate between stunted (short, with relatively normal weight for height) and wasted (relatively normal height, with low weight for height) children. However, it requires *two* items of equipment—the Thinness Chart and weighing scales—and the education and literacy (numeracy) to be able to use them in a correct sequence. Confusion may also arise because red (indicating thinness) is on a *higher* level than other colors, in contrast to the fact that red often represents the *lower* levels used in multiline weight charts and in arm circumference tapes. This chart is more useful for screening than for detailed monitoring as changes can only be detected over a prolonged period, probably 6 months.

RECORDING RESULTS

Weights

The adequacy of a child's weight can be assessed in two ways.

1. *Single Weight.* First visit or after prolonged absence, in relation to lines on growth chart or to weight reference data, such as the U.S. National Center for Health Statistics (NCHS) figures (Hamill et al., 1979), which are often used because of being internationally available and acceptable by WHO as appropriate for young children in most genetic groups. However, it must be stressed that a single measurement is not "monitoring." If it is all that is available, the approximate information obtained needs to be used cautiously and combined with other knowledge, such as the child's general appearance and clinical history.

2. *Serial Weights.* Two, or preferably three, consecutive weighings at appropriate intervals for the child's age can be plotted on the growth chart and the slope of the line made by joining these points looked at to indicate *satisfactory growth* (adequate gain) or *unsatisfactory growth* (inadequate gain, no gain, or loss). Alternatively, serial measurements can be recorded in "weight boxes," as have been used in the Philippines (Griffiths, 1981b) (Fig. 2-16) or devised by Essex and Gosling (1987) and termed "growth action records" (Fig. 2-17). These may be easier for community health workers in recording growth, but they lack the potential visual educational values of the altered slope of a child's growth line on a weight chart.

Nowadays, almost all graphs are in the metric system. Unfortunately, some have a metric scale on the left with a parallel scale on the right side in pounds and ounces. This is obviously undesirable and confusing. Alternatively, the Salter metric scale can be modified by sticking on an appropriate thin cardboard dial showing pounds and ounces. Curiously, this has been the practice in Guatemala. Also, in the English-speaking Caribbean and certain Latin American countries (such as Colombia), some scales are still in pounds. They badly need replacement with matching metric scales and graphs.

In a very few countries, the graphs read from right to left. This is so in the Maldive Islands in accordance with their written language. However, most Arab countries have left-to-right graphs.

Weight Graphs (Charts)

At least five main types of "take-home" weight charts or graphs are in use or under trial in different parts of the world. All have advantages and potential difficulties. All need to be used mainly to monitor growth—that is, weight increase with time as shown by the slope of the weights charted on the graph. Some charts also attempt to categorize children who are significantly below weight.

Two-Line Graph (Figs. 2-7a and 2-7b)

This is the classical Morley-WHO "Road to Health Chart" [upper reference line fiftieth NCHS centile[1] for boys, and lower reference line third centile (*approximately* 80%, or −2 SD; SD is standard deviation) for girls]. Most, but not all, healthy children will have growth curves between these lines. Also, as stressed elsewhere, it is the slope of the curve that is the main concern, and the three main categories of slope are usually illustrated on the card pictorially (upward = growth, flat = no growth, downward = weight loss).

Modified Two-Line Graph

One or two modifications may be made.

- Dotted lines or colored bands can be included between the two main reference lines, forming "channels" following the slope of the main curve, and/or
- A dotted line can be included below the lower reference line (often at 70% or −3 SD) to indicate very low weight or emergency weight level.

Also, additional dotted lines between the two reference lines can give additional channels (Fig. 2-8). Five extra dotted lines between the two main refer-

---

1. Recent work in many parts of the world has shown differences in growth in breastfed compared with bottle-fed babies. Breastfed babies show a first trimester growth spurt, followed by a normal physiological growth deceleration. This needs to be taken into account in assessing growth. There is the likelihood that modified lines may be used in future growth charts prepared specifically for breastfed infants.

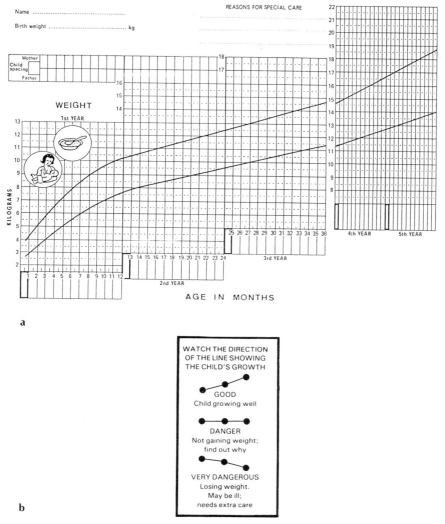

Figure 2-7 (a) WHO two-line road-to-health chart (sexes combined) (WHO, 1978b). Normal growth parallels the growth lines; most children's weights will be between the two lines. (b) WHO two-line road-to-health chart (WHO, 1978b); indicative growth lines.

ences lines are both practicable and mathematically understandable, as each dotted line would then represent −0.33 SD (e.g., from the median to −2 SD, or 100% to 80%). If culturally appropriate and economically feasible, the six channels could be graded downward by shading a single culturally appropriate color from darker to lighter (or from lighter to darker, if shown to be more understandable locally). In countries where obesity in young children is a prob-

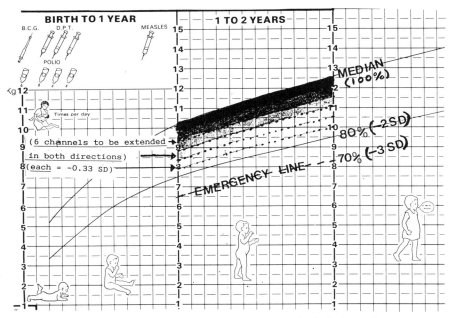

Figure 2-8 Modified two-line growth chart with (a) shaded channels at 0.33 SD (standard deviation) intervals between main lines, and (b) lower dotted line (emergency line) (-3SD).

lem, higher overweight dotted lines can be included at 120% (or +2 SD) and above, if felt useful.

If *five* additional dotted lines are introduced between the two main reference lines at −0.33 SD intervals, this would lead to *six* appropriately shaded channels. This could be of assistance in guiding recognition of different levels of satisfactory or unsatisfactory growth (p. 42–44).

Inadequate weight gain could be defined as a child growing very slowly, but moving to *one channel lower* in *1 month* in the first 6 months of life, in *2 months* from 6 to 12 months, and in *3 months* in the second and third year. These simple definitions are speculative, need further investigation in practice, and may need modification.

Multiline Charts (Figs. 2-9 and 2-10)

Various reference lines may be included below the median (labeled 100%). For example, 100%, 90%, 75%, and 60% (the original classical Gómez Classification, which is still used in some countries; Gómez et al., 1956); or 100%, 80%, and 60% (Jelliffe, 1966).

The lines on such charts may differ in some countries. For example, the Indian Pediatric Association used 80% of the Harvard reference level as their practical median (or 100%). This may be considered necessary if most children do not "fit" on a regular chart. However, this has the risk of becoming per-

Fig. I.2.9 Multi Line Chart (100%, 80%, 60%)

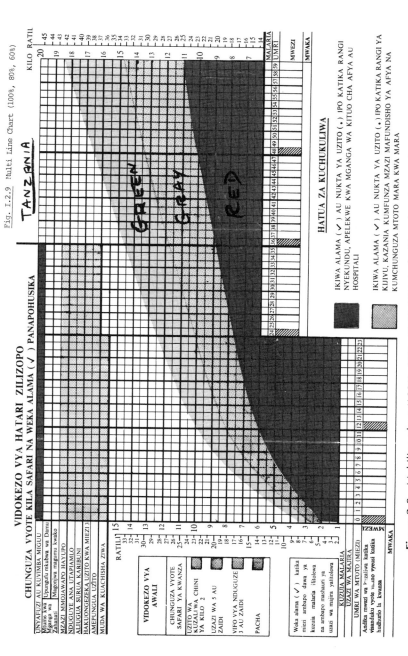

Figure 2-9 Multiline chart (100%, 80%, 60%). (Original with colored zones.)

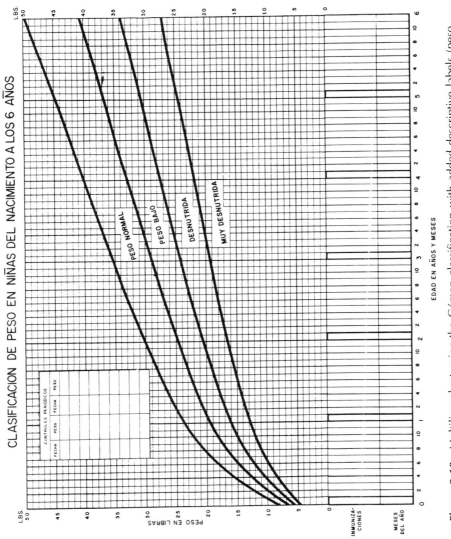

Figure 2-10 Multiline chart using the Gómez classification with added descriptive labels (*peso bajo*: low weight, etc.) (Colombia).

petuated and labeling as normal some who are malnourished and at higher risk of serious infection. If used, it must be constantly recalled that these modifications are interim. This is difficult to do, as such charts become widely used and thus are considered normal for the area. Revision is needed at intervals of not more than 5 years. However, if such modification is done, it is better and simpler that the lines should be selected, at percent levels of NCHS. This permits greater comparability and upward movement of the lines as the nutritional level of children in the community improves.

The areas between the different lines are often colored (Fig. 2-9) and sometimes also labeled low weight, malnourished, and so forth. As with the two-line charts, these can also have dotted lines or shaded colored bands to give channels between the main lines. Whenever color is used, this should be culturally appropriate. For example, in Indonesia, green symbolizes health and yellow illness; in different countries such as China and Ecuador, red indicates wellness.

The disadvantage of multiline charts is that they tend to focus exclusive attention on categorization or classification—that is, current nutritional assessment—and can distract attention from observation of the child's growth. This is accentuated if the areas between the lines are colored and/or labeled with descriptive labels such as normal, low, malnourished, or very malnourished (Fig. 2-10).

Single-Line Graphs

In a small number of countries, including Zimbabwe and the Dominican Republic (Fig. 2-11), a single-line growth chart is used. The line is often the −2 SD (approximately 80%). This has the advantage of simplicity, as an upper line is not of much significance in practice, and the focus should be on the child's growth *curve*. Difficulties in the Dominican Republic graph include the 500-g markings together with the adjacent levels in kilograms and pounds, and the extension of the chart for children up to 5 years of age.

Multichannel Graphs

Recently, Burns, Carrière, and Rohde (1988) devised a logical growth chart designed exclusively to facilitate recognition of early evidence of slowing of growth (Fig. 2-12). This is a multichannel ''rainbow'' graph with 15 colored channels, but with no lines indicating percentages or statistically defined levels (standard deviations or centiles).

The multichannel chart is based on the following attributes (Burns, Carrière, & Rohde, 1988).

1. *Linear accentuation should be longest* in the vertical scale to demonstrate the rising curve of growth and thereby clearly indicate when an inadequate rise in line represents a faltering growth. Design should carefully employ the entire vertical range available to accentuate the rise associated with growth.

2. *A key to trend lines* should be prominently displayed accentuating normal, flat, and decreasing growth lines. This should be the predominant interpretation

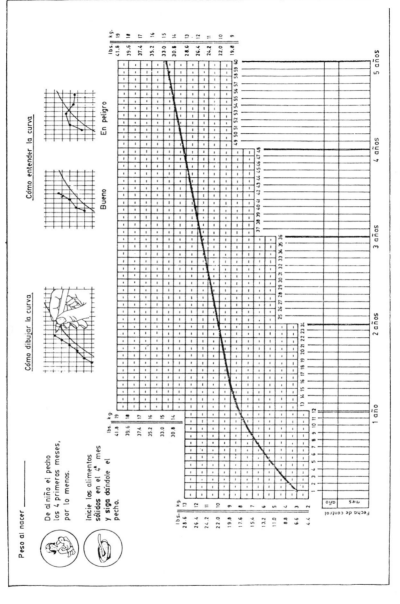

Figure 2-11 Single-line weight chart (third centile) (Dominican Republic).

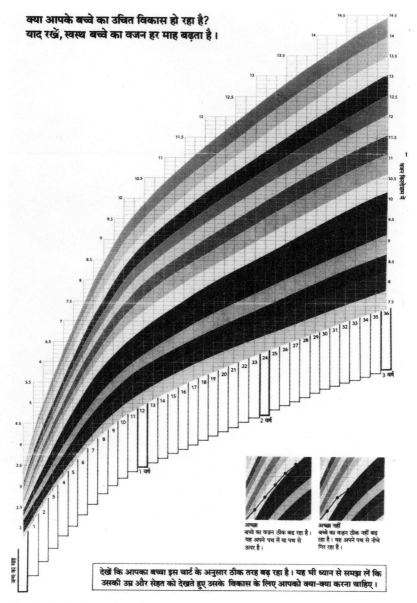

Figure 2-12 Multichannel rainbow growth chart (Burns, Carrière & Rohde, 1988). Channels are in different vivid colors and chart is tall to assist in detecting abnormal growth (Indian version).

of the card, not determination of nutritional categories. Trend lines should emphasize month-by-month growth trends, not long-term trends.

3. *Narrow lightly colored or shaded bands may assist in the identification of normal trend lines.* These should not be clearly delineated as nutritional categories but only represent a family of curves that will show the normal direction of growth in children in a normal population.

4. *Accuracy of plotting is facilitated by:* (a) Offset of the month labels so that they appear at the bottom of vertical month lines, each properly numbered; (b) Division of kilogram, 500-g, and 100-g lines in different colors or by other means (circles). One hundred-gram divisions are essential as normal monthly weight gain beyond 12 months of age is less than 200 g; (c) Position of month label boxes rising toward the right side of the chart, minimizing distance to plot. Vertical lines delineating months should arise from the center of the month label box in order to make the choice of which vertical line represents the particular month entirely unambiguous; and (d) Kilogram numbers placed at intervals across the face of the chart to avoid the necessity of reading across from the lateral margin of the card.

5. *The card should be attractive, using color printing and material that is durable.* This would enhance the inherent value of the card to the mother as well as to the health worker and is well worth the added investment.

6. *Age range should be limited to less than 3 years of age* and consideration given in different programs to a less than 2 years or even an 18 months age limit. This will further accentuate the period of maximal growth and early growth faltering in the child, particularly the importance of the introduction of weaning foods in a timely way.

7. *Nutritional status category.* The major impediment to effective use of growth cards for monitoring the trend of growth (in contrast to a tool for periodic nutritional assessment) is the presence of multiple lines corresponding to cut off points for nutritional categories. Serious consideration should be given to the elimination of such clear lines on the chart and their replacement by trend lines shown by shading the color bands in the printing process. Plastic overlay charts could then be used by health workers who are attempting to screen children by determining the nutritional status and percentages of standards as a means of identifying high-risk children to receive nutritional supplements.

Recently, Griffiths (1987, 1988) has introduced the "Bubble Chart" (Fig. 2-13), which is taller and makes changes in growth lines more obvious and is easier to plot weights. It has recently been used successfully in several countries (Griffiths & Berg, 1989).

Cards (Health or Wellness Records). Great variation exists between cards with regard to details, including their size (often 21 cm × 30 cm), the number of years covered, the space (distance) between "month lines" (often 0.5 cm horizontally) and between kilogram levels (often 1 cm vertically), the bottom of the graph (flat or stepped), and the repetition of weight figures on the vertical lines at the beginning of each year.

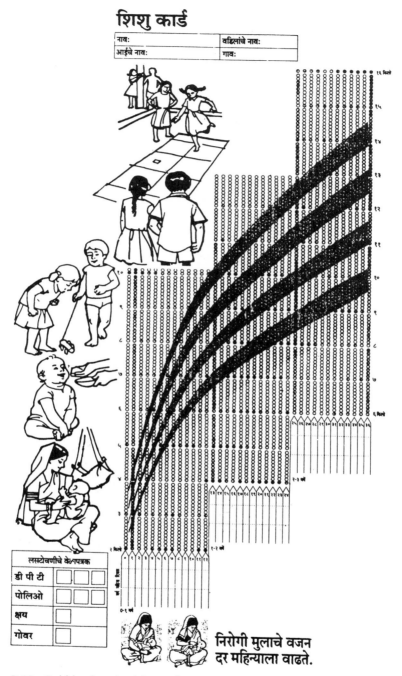

Figure 2-13 Bubble chart (weight) (Indian version) (Griffiths, 1987 & 1988). Child's weight can be plotted more easily as the "bubbles" are at 100-g intervals. Also, the tall vertical axis makes it easier to detect flattening of growth curves. (Original with colored zones.)

Such cards are usually issued free but, in some countries, a very small price has been charged to increase their significance in the mother's eyes and as a token entry ticket to the clinic (Chaudhuri, 1988). This type of chart is almost always designed to be retained by mothers, often in a plastic container in order to keep them clean. To eliminate the cost of the plastic container (which may be used instead by mothers for other purposes), cards made of sturdy, cleanable, waterproof plasticized paper are being tried out. Taller cards (with a higher vertical axis) will enable flattening of growth curves to be detected more easily, as with the multichannel Rainbow Chart (Fig. 2-12) and the Bubble Chart (Fig. 2-13). Larger charts have weight graphs that may be easier to understand and certainly make within-month plotting (i.e., earlier or later) more possible. However, a large chart will be difficult to carry and may be more easily bent or damaged.

A wide range of other information may be included in different ways on the front and/or back of the card, such as:

1. A listing of reasons for special care (locally important risk factors).
2. Records of other procedures or practices, such as immunizations, antimalarial medicine, diet being taken, or family planning methods used.
3. Written and visual information, reminders, and advice on a variety of topics, including the date recommended for the next visit and items mentioned in point 2.
4. Advertisements for commercial products should not be included (unless congruent with health objectives).

The educational potential of a home-based card is often underappreciated. This needs to be a well-designed communications strategy designed with full involvement of the population served (Griffiths, 1988). This has also been emphasized recently by Burns and Rohde (1988).

A carefully designed growth chart can be one of the most powerful education tools in nutrition and health. No other record is generally given to the mother and can so attractively display the growth and health of her child. Careful consideration of each element of a card, particularly those fostering an understanding and appreciation of growth, but also the other messages and records to be included, is an imperative to make the investment in this communication tool a truly effective one. Growth card design has too long followed the simple graphic display found in pediatric textbooks or in hospital charts the world over. When viewed as an educational tool that will be valued and retained by the mother, one can see that the design of growth cards is one of the most important elements of the successful growth monitoring and promotion program.

If not weighed from birth, the child's age may be uncertain or unknown. The construction of a local calendar of events may be needed to assess the age (Jelliffe & Jelliffe, 1990).

The usefulness of such home-based child's cards (HBCR) is not only of potential educational value for parents. The cards can also be an informative record if the child is hospitalized or moving elsewhere. They have therefore been aptly termed "child health passports" (Wit et al., 1984).

Largely underappreciated in the English language literature is the fact that in Francophone countries, such as those in West Africa, various modifications of the *carnet de santé* (health booklet), distributed to all mothers at delivery in France,[2] are employed. All include an extensive range of information on pregnancy, growth in early childhood (usually to be recorded graphically) (Fig. 2-14), immunizations, advice of diet, notes on treatment, and so forth. Problems with cost of production and distribution must be considered. A token, nominal charge is made in some countries, not to cover the cost, but to increase the importance and value in mothers' minds.

Assistance with Weight Plotting. In view of the difficulties with plotting weights on graphs, the Bubble Chart and the TALC scale, which has a simple, direct plotting device as one practical innovation, are undergoing field trials in various parts of the world. Promising reports with the TALC scale have been observed in some African countries, such as Sierra Leone and Liberia.

Assuming that some form of graphic weight chart will be used indefinitely for the foreseeable future in many countries, a "Right-Way Weight Plotter" card has been suggested as a simple aid (Fig. 2-15a), with assistance on the back (Right-Way Weight Assessor) to help in gauging adequacy of weight gain from the *slopes* of the growth lines (Fig. 2-15b). Alterations will be required to suit local needs and experience. This weight plotter is a further adaptation of the method advocated by Morley and Woodland (1979) using a square-edged piece of paper.

Weight Boxes. To avoid problems with plotting weights on graphs, the use of weight boxes has been suggested in the Philippines (Fig. 2-16) and by Essex and Gosling (1987) (growth action records) (Fig. 2-17). Both avoid the need for any understanding of graphs and clearly indicate significantly low weight levels. Neither seems to have as much potential visual impact as does a satisfactory or unsatisfactory growth curve. They need further trial in appropriate circumstances.

Arm Circumference. If this method is used, particularly during home visiting, an insertion arm tape (Zerfas, 1975) has been devised that is graduated in centimeters *and* color coded, or just color coded (Fig. 2-18a) (Jelliffe & Jelliffe, 1989). In this case, any record card used should be such that health workers can either plot the arm circumference by color or in centimeters. A preliminary version of this type of color tape was introduced and used successfully in Burkina Faso (Zeitlin et al., 1982).

2. Details of the *carnet de santé* as used in France were given by Sempé and Masse (1965) and by Sénécal and Roussey (1976). In the United Kingdom, various home-based health booklets are used in different parts of the country, but these vary from area to area (Lakhani et al., 1984). A similar "Health Booklet" *(Bukana)* is under trial in Lesotho in southern Africa (Moteetee, 1989).

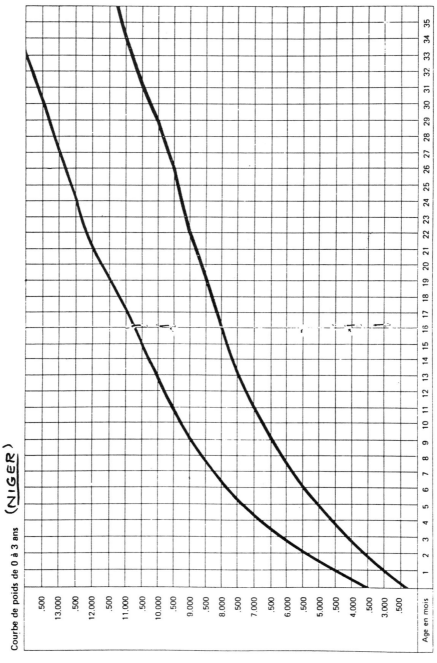

Figure 2-14 *Carnet de santé* (health booklet) showing two-line growth curves (Niger).

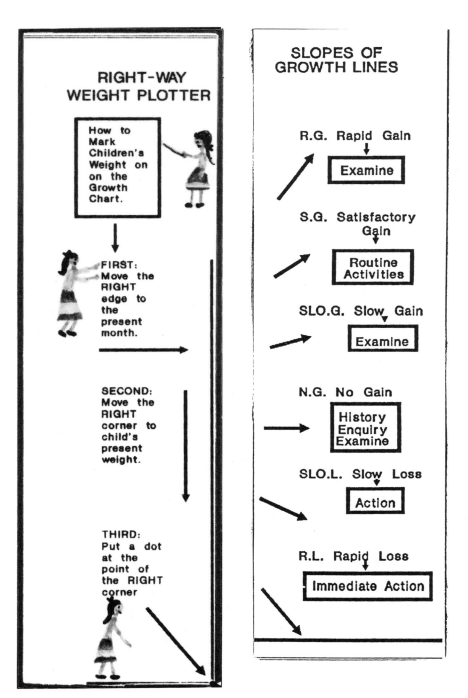

Figure 2-15 (a) Right-way weight plotter. (b) Right-way weight assessor (reverse side of plotter), using slopes of growth lines.

Name ______________________
Date of Birth ______________________

PHILIPPINE NUTRITION PROGRAM

NUTRITION HEALTH CHART FOR BABIES

PROVINCE: ______________________
MUNICIPALITY: ______________________
BARANGAY: ______________________

	MONTH	Birth-month	1	2	3	4	5	6	7	8	9	10	11	12	13	14	15	16	17	18
	WEIGHT (Kg)																			
	NUTRITION LEVEL	(PLOT MONTHLY WEIGHT IN CORRECT BLOCK TO DETERMINE NUTRITION LEVEL)																		
	1 HEALTHY	3.1	3.8	4.5	5.1	5.7	6.2	6.7	7.1	7.6	8.0	8.3	8.6	8.9	9.1	9.3	9.5	9.7	9.9	10.1
MILDLY MALNOURISHED	2	2.9	3.6	4.2	4.8	5.4	5.9	6.3	6.7	7.1	7.6	7.8	8.2	8.4	8.6	8.8	9.0	9.2	9.4	9.5
	3	2.7	3.4	4.0	4.6	5.0	5.5	5.9	6.3	6.7	7.1	7.4	7.7	7.9	8.1	8.2	8.5	8.6	8.8	9.0
	4	2.6	3.2	3.8	4.3	4.7	5.2	5.6	5.9	6.3	6.7	6.9	7.2	7.4	7.6	7.7	8.0	8.1	8.2	8.4
MODERATELY MALNOURISHED	5	2.4	2.9	3.5	4.0	4.4	4.8	5.2	5.5	5.9	6.2	6.4	6.7	6.9	7.1	7.2	7.4	7.6	7.7	7.8
	6	2.2	2.7	3.2	3.7	4.1	4.5	4.8	5.1	5.5	5.8	6.0	6.2	6.4	6.6	6.7	6.9	7.0	7.2	7.3
	7	2.0	2.5	3.0	3.4	3.8	4.1	4.4	4.7	5.0	5.3	5.5	5.8	5.9	6.1	6.2	6.4	6.5	6.6	6.7
SEVERLY MALNOURISHED	8	1.9	2.3	2.8	3.1	3.5	3.8	4.1	4.3	4.6	4.9	5.1	5.3	5.4	5.6	5.7	5.8	5.9	6.1	6.2
	9	1.7	2.1	2.2	2.8	3.2	3.4	3.7	4.0	4.2	4.6	4.6	4.8	5.0	5.1	5.2	5.3	5.4	5.5	5.6
	10																			

Philippine Growth Table USAID Mission

Figure 2-16 Nutrition health chart: weight boxes (Philippines). Child's weight indicated in appropriate box for month of age, suggesting categorization (moderately malnourished, etc.). Increases or decreases in weight can be observed in rise or fall in level of boxes filled.

GROWTH ACTION RECORD

Child's name . . . . Date of birth . . . .
Mother's name . . . . Address . . . .
Father's name . . . . Village . . . .

VACCINATIONS

☐ BCG
☐ DPT, Polio
☐ Measles

ACTIONS

RA PE	Routine activities Praise and encourage
FF	More frequent followup
AP	Action package
HV	Home visit
R	Refer to health centre

EXTRA CARE BABIES

☐	Low birth weight	History of malnutrition
☐	Bottle feeding	One parent only
☐	Unvaccinated	Measles
☐	Twins	Whooping cough
☐	Orphan	Frequent diarrhoea
☐	Previous infant death	

Circle next visit ○   Mark failure to attend ⊗

FIRST YEAR   SECOND YEAR   THIRD YEAR

AGE months	BIRTH	1	2	3	4	5	6	7	8	9	10	11	12	13	14	15	16	17	18	19	20	21	22	23	24	25	26	27	28	29	30	31	32	33	34	35	36
MONTHS		Attend monthly									Attend every 2 months									Attend every 6 months																	
WEIGHT kgs.																																						
Danger	2 5	2 9	3 5	4 0	4 6	5 1	5 5	5 9	6 4	6 8	7 1	7 4	7 7	7 9	8 1	8 3	8 4	8 6	8 7	8 8	9 0	9 2	9 3	9 4	9 6	9 7	9 8	10 0	10 2	10 3	10 5	10 7	10 8	11 0	11 1	11 2	11 4
Emergency	1 8	1 9	2 3	2 6	3 0	3 3	3 6	3 8	4 2	4 7	5 5	5 7	6 0	6 3	6 5	6 6	6 7	6 8	7 0	7 2	7 5	7 7	7 8	7 9	8 0	8 2	8 3	8 5	8 7	8 8	9 0	9 2	9 3	9 5	9 7	9 8	10 0
ACTIONS																																						

Figure 2-17 Growth action record (Essex & Gosling, 1987). Child's weight is entered in box beneath the appropriate month, with lower boxes indicating danger or emergency.

65

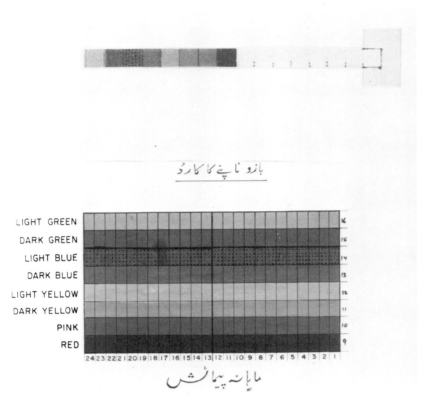

بازو ناپنے كا كارڈ

LIGHT GREEN	۱۶
DARK GREEN	۱۵
LIGHT BLUE	۱۴
DARK BLUE	۱۳
LIGHT YELLOW	۱۲
DARK YELLOW	۱۱
PINK	۱۰
RED	۹

24 23 22 21 20 19 18 17 16 15 14 13 12 11 10 9 8 7 6 5 4 3 2 1

ماہانہ پیمائش

Figure 2-18 Growth maintenance (a) arm insertion tape and (b) color-coded record; designed for use by illiterate community health workers with no knowledge of graphing; figures on chart indicate *attendance* (1 = first time, 4 = fourth time, etc.), *not* the child's age. The main objective is to maintain the arm circumference at or above the 15-cm level or other locally defined level. (Trial version, Pakistan reading from right to left.)

A growth maintenance multicolor arm tape (Fig. 2-18b) needs further testing and modification as regards usefulness in an approximate monitoring process instead of in screening and for its practical value for illiterate community health workers. As noted elsewhere, such an instrument is cheap and easily portable, but needs to be considered for trying to insure growth *maintenance* rather than growth increase after reaching the local normal level for 1- to 4-year-old children—often 16 cm. The method does not have the same potential as the *increasing* growth shown on a weight graph. The objective is to *maintain* the arm circumference at a satisfactory level.

3

Varying Circumstances, Varying Systems

COMMON VARIABLES

Effective, practical growth monitoring systems need to take into account many environmental, demographic, health, educational, cultural, and financial considerations. These can vary greatly in different countries, and even in different areas of some countries.

Some of the more important variations are listed next; they relate especially to feasible activities of community health workers as part of primary health services. These cadres will usually be expected to undertake most growth monitoring in less technically developed countries, either at village clinics or centers, during home visits, or at rallies or gatherings of children at more prolonged intervals.

1. Environmental and Demographic Variables.
   a. Size of the area served.
   b. Numbers of people served, particularly young children.
   c. Nearness of clinic to homes (distance time required for visit).
   d. Distribution of houses (villages, scattered dwellings, etc.).
   e. Accessibility for home visiting (terrain, roads, and weather).
2. Health of Children.
   a. Prevalence of important preventable infections in young children.
   b. Commonest forms of childhood malnutrition, including age incidence and most frequent causes.
3. Health Services.
   a. Type, extent, nearness, and real level of activities of other health service units (health clinics, hospitals).
   b. Health manpower: existing, planned, and numbers of training establishments.
   c. Training of community health workers: time, content, practicality.
   d. Actual supervision of community health workers.
4. Educational.
   a. Literacy rate, including level of literacy.
   b. Familiarity with decimal system.

    c. Pictorial and graphic literacy.

    d. Availability of schools.

    e. Preference, regarding community health workers: age (old versus young), sex, educated, married, with own children.

5. Cultural.

    a. Eagerness or unwillingness to have young children weighed.

    b. Local methods of recognizing growth or thinness.

    c. Restrictions on female workers' activities (e.g., home visiting).

    d. Understanding reading of circular dial on weighing scale.

    e. Ability to understand a graph and to plot on it.

6. Financial.

    a. National health budget (especially amount for all primary health care activities and percent of budget available for limited period from donor agencies).

    b. Cost of equipment: (1) Scales (including repairs and replacement); (2) Clinic cards, preferably Home-Based Child Records (HBCR), including a method of recording weight, usually a graph; (3) Community health workers salaries (or other remuneration); (4) Transport (type needed, fuel, drivers' salaries, repairs).

MAIN VARIABLES

The variations just listed influence the feasibility of using a particular growth monitoring system in many interacting ways. The following points are especially important:

General Educational Level and Training of Community Health Workers

In various countries, *different individuals are responsible for growth monitoring.* These can vary from trained nurses (or occasionally physicians), to often briefly trained, semiliterate workers (community health workers) selected by the village or community itself and, in a very few places, to mothers themselves or to older siblings (schoolchildren).

In practice, most growth monitoring will be undertaken by community health workers, who vary greatly in background, general education, and special training for primary health care activities. With the great variation in length (a few days to several months), type, and relevance of training and of field circumstances, considerable differences must be expected in the capabilities and functions of community health workers in different countries or areas. For example, the level of general education can influence the ability to weigh accurately, to plot the results on a weight chart and, especially, to interpret the growth lines of children on such charts and to judge appropriate actions.

Understandability by mothers seems to vary greatly. In a project in Indonesia, mothers were shown to be able to weigh young children and plot the results

(Rohde et al., 1979). In the Jamkhed Project in India, Arole (1988) was of the opinion that illiterate mothers understood the meaning of growth better than literate women from the same area. In Jamaica (Brunetto & Pearson 1987), Papua-New Guinea (Forsyth, 1984), Tamil Nadu, India (Srilatha, 1986), and elsewhere, difficulties have been encountered with mothers' understanding and with the usefulness of the weight graph as an educational tool. On the other hand, it has been stressed by Hendrata and Rohde (1988 and previously) that this may be more a reflection of the training and understanding of community health workers and their ability to communicate effectively with mothers and involve them in practically the whole process. This is more likely to be achievable in relatively small, well-supervised pilot projects than when replicated in very large national populations.

Technical Considerations

These will include the *type of scale* and *weight charts* (or other record) to be used, as outlined earlier. These is considerable variation in the *age range included* in different growth charts from 0 to 3 years up to 0 to 7 years. As a generalization, there seems to be a trend toward covering only the first 2 to 3 years. This includes both the time when growth is often optimal (0 months to 4 to 6 months) and positive reinforcement and preventive health measures can be introduced (including advice on the introduction of semisolid foods in the second semester, immunization, etc.) and also the time span when malnutrition most often occurs (e.g., the second and third years).

The suggested *frequency of weighing* advised also differs. Ideally, in most circumstances, weighing should be monthly through the first 3 years, preferably commencing at or shortly after birth. Currently, WHO (1986) recommends the following: once monthly, first year; twice monthly, second year; and three times monthly, third year. In addition, and from a practical point of view, weighing and recording should be carried out any time a child attends a clinic or is visited at home.

As a means of *promoting* good growth, weighing should be started at birth and continued frequently (at least monthly) during the first 6 months. As growth during this period is usually good in breastfed babies, this enables positive reinforcement (praise) to be given to the mother, making suggestions and guidance concerning the introduction of other complementary foods at an appropriate time more likely to be followed (Hendrata & Rohde, 1988) and satisfactory growth continued or promoted after this. Difficulties may include cultural anxieties (such as vulnerability of small babies to the "Evil Eye"), logistic problems in weighing at or near birth, the possible need for an additional, more accurate method for weighing young babies, and the fact that frequent weighing will also need to be targeted to the age range (often 1 to 2 or 3 years), when growth failure is known to be more common in the particular community. As with other considerations, decisions have to be made related to resources, problems, and purposes.

Methods of *identifying unsatisfactory growth* will vary with circumstances, but with *graphic recording* will mainly be done by observing the slope of the growth line made by joining the dots recorded at two or preferably three *serial weighings* made at appropriate intervals of the child's age *or,* with much less significance, the position on the graph of a *single weight recording.* This would be when a child attends a clinic or center for the first time or after a prolonged period.

Individual variation is another consideration in interpreting growth curves of different children. Sometimes, lower weight levels may have a specific identifiable reason, as with a baby with a low birth weight or with small parents. It must be appreciated that growth is more rapid in the earlier months of infancy than later. Unsatisfactory weight gain is of greater significance in the young baby, especially during the first months of life.

Additionally, the growth of a healthy young child never follows a completely smooth, uninterrupted weight curve. Irregular growth can occur normally, and some minor changes in weight can depend on whether the child has been fed recently. Sudden serious alterations can, of course, be due to diarrheal dehydration or edema.

Careful longitudinal weight charting of well-nourished young children in the United Kingdom and Hong Kong also showed upward or downward "crossing or centiles" in small, but significant, percentages (Davies & Leung, 1984). However, in poorly nourished child populations in less technically developed countries, where widespread infections are usual, even lesser degrees of unsatisfactory weight gain need to be viewed as potentially serious, accompanied by a careful history from the mother and general examination of the infant.

Time and motion considerations have to be considered with regard to the usual *numbers of young children* attending each session, taking into consideration the *number of staff* and *their other duties,* the *time taken to weigh* and explain the child's growth line to the mother, and the *time taken for other routine activities* (such as noting new "risk" factors, recording infant feeding and family planning practices, immunizations given, and advising on feeding and other health concerns), and *time for special activities,* such as limited treatments [especially oral rehydration (ORT)], the issue and explanation of supplementary foods or nutrients (e.g., vitamin A, when needed and if available), and immunization, if feasible. The question of budgeting of time in overcrowded circumstances is often not appreciated. This is especially the case if training is undertaken by different teachers who "specialize" in one aspect of a child survival program. Each may narrowly emphasize important details needed of the community health workers in that particular task without considering the range and time required for other expected duties.

Distances and Support Services

Key concerns for the community health worker's work include *distances and difficulty of travel* by the worker for follow-up or increased home visits and/or, alternatively, regular or increased visits by mothers (or parents) to the community health workers clinic. The need for follow-up or extra visits may be indicated by a recording system at the clinic to identify the most underprivileged and the "defaulters" when they fail to attend.

Insuring that the most needy are included may require special attention, particularly in communities with distant, scattered dwellings and rough terrain. For example, in an area in the Himalayas, a system termed "health shepherding" has been used, particularly based on home visits and referral of children at risk (Lankester, 1988).

Referral may also be limited by the cost, distance, infrequency of transport and difficulty of travel to a health center or hospital. In addition, in some areas health centers and hospitals are themselves so swamped that the services may be little or no better than can be provided by the community health workers.

Supervision and in-service training are important aspects needed for effective community health workers performance. Both are frequently inadequate. Supervision is often limited and perfunctory. It can sometimes become non-supportive and a disciplinary inspection. Rather, it needs to be helpful and educational, but again from a practical viewpoint the feasibility and frequency necessarily varies greatly with distances to be traveled and available manpower.

Community Involvement and Organization

This will vary with different circumstances, including traditional cultural practices, such as ancient built-in systems involving discussion, consensus, and group support, local methods of recognizing growth (i.e., bangles or limb beads that are too tight, the need for larger clothes), and the degree of success of the community health workers or other community representatives (such as parent-teacher groups or older schoolchildren) in involving mothers in all growth monitoring activities, including weighing, plotting, interpreting results for appropriate action (decision making), and training other mothers.

Newer additional methods involving mothers can be undertaken in a variety of ways, such as focus group interviews (Manoff, 1985; Scrimshaw & Hurtado, 1987) (Appendix C) or more extensive discussions.

CONTRASTING EXAMPLES

A great variety of successful systems have evolved in different parts of the world. Comparative descriptions of different programs in the Dominican Republic, Thailand, Indonesia, and Tamil Nadu, India, are given later (Appendix G). As can be seen, the level of training, the numbers of workers, and the sequence and equipment used vary greatly, as does the degree of community involvement and participation.

4

Methods of Assessment

> All over Africa, children are weighed and measured while mothers look on with varying degrees of interest and understanding, and the health staff then says a few words and records the measurements on growth cards and perhaps tally sheets. . . . Even if the technique of the procedure is done correctly, the advice that follows on management is neither adequate nor helpful.
>
> Editorial, *East African Medical Journal* (1986)

ADEQUACY OF GROWTH

Comparison with Standard Figures

In practice, the growth of young children is usually judged by observing weight change. Weight gain over a defined period can be compared with average figures for children of that age. Even so, there are problems, since figures given by different authors vary to some extent and may be categorized as normal or average, minimum, or inadequate for varying periods of time, for example, 1, 2, or 3 months. One simplified list is given in Table 4-1. The method requires subtraction and lacks a visual message for community health workers and mothers. As experience has shown, inaccurately taken weights recorded in this way are most often written down as an ill-understood ritual, without enthusiasm, interest, or action, if any is indicated.

Growth Charts

The adequacy of growth is usually estimated by the slope on a graph of the line made by joining two or preferably three weight recordings plotted at what are judged to be appropriate intervals for young children of different ages.

Table 4-1 Inadequate weight gain levels

Age	Weight gain	Time
0–12 months	330 grams or less	one month
1–2 years	470 grams or less	2 months
2–3 years	500 grams or less	3 months

Three slopes are commonly considered—upward, flat, and downward (Morley, 1968). As noted earlier, however, the two-line WHO-Morley type Road to Health Chart can be modified with six channels between the main lines and an "emergency" or "very low weight line" below (Fig. 4-1). On this chart, most but not all nonmalnourished children will show growth between the two main lines, and from the slope of an individual child's plotted "growth line" various "growth categories" may be considered.

- *Upward*

  RG   = rapid gain, into higher channel
  SG   = satisfactory gain, in same channel
  Slo.G = slow gain, weight increasing, but into lower channels

- *Flat*

  NG   = no gain

- *Downward*

  Slo.L = slow loss
  RL   = rapid loss

The number of growth categories selected in practice depends on the ease of definition for the community health workers and their actual functional significance in terms of realistic action that may be feasible. In practice, only *two main categories* need to be recognized initially, although different actions are needed for some subcategories indicated. These two categories are:

1. *Satisfactory growth:* RG (rapid gain), SG (satisfactory gain).
2. *Unsatisfactory growth:* Slo.G (slow gain), NG (no gain), Slo.L (slow loss), RL (rapid loss).

Various difficulties exist with this classification. Firstly, "slow weight gain" (Slo.G) with *gradually* increasing weight, but nevertheless falling into lower growth channels, needs to be defined and explained in an understandable way for the community health workers. This may be done by a fall in a stated number of channels (if such are present on the graph) as suggested earlier, or by visual comparison of the slope with lines indicating slow gain included on the chart or on the reverse side of the Right-Way Weight Plotter (Figs. 2-15*a* and 2.15*b*.) Details need to be decided to suit local conditions.

Second, with all charts, it is important that weight loss, failure to gain, or inadequate weight gain *above* the upper line be recognized as equally significant as similar changes lower on the graph.

Nevertheless, initial weights or curves commencing just below the lower line need special attention. This may be abnormal or within normal limits as, for example, in children with small parents or with a low birth weight. Inquiry should be made about *general history* from the mother, including birth weight, size of parents, whether twins, and so on, *feeding history,* including breast-feeding and weaning diet, *symptoms* and *signs of infections,* and *examination*

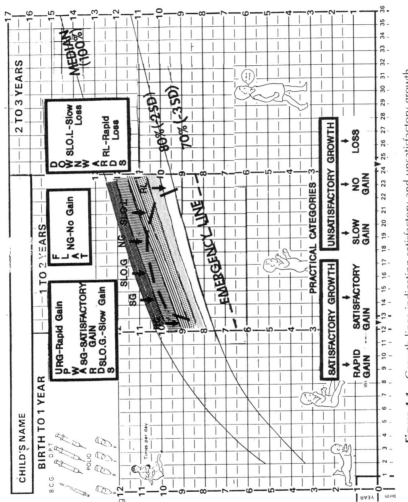

Figure 4-1 Growth lines indicating satisfactory and unsatisfactory growth.

to judge "general appearance" and to identify certain more obvious clinical signs. This must be followed by *careful attention at regular attendances* at clinics or centers (or home visits) to insure satisfactory subsequent catch-up weight gain.

Last, a very rapid increase in weight needs to take into account the possibility of the development of edema. Conversely, a rapid fall must bear in mind the possibility of diarrheal dehydration.

Position on Growth Chart

If a "very low weight" or "emergency" line (often at 70% or −3 SD) is included in the graph, this may be helpful to the community health workers as one immediate and clear indication for urgent action. This will usually be because a single measurement has been made at the first attendance or, alternatively, following a prolonged period of nonattendance.

Once again, it must be stressed that monitoring by serial weighing, followed by prompt interpretation and action, is the goal. Nevertheless, occasionally a single measurement may be all that is available and can sometimes be helpful, but it must be interpreted with much caution.

Developing decision diagrams. Decision diagrams (flowcharts) or decision lists can be useful in suggesting interpretations and actions. Those given in this book are sometimes designed in a seemingly logical sequence (decision diagram) and are sometimes designed to suggest alternatives (decision list). These are only general examples, and relevant decision diagrams and lists must be prepared to suit local circumstances. Also, as noted later, they may occasionally be available in simplified forms for guidance for literate community health workers in a clinic or other primary health care setting. More usually, they can be employed in a simplified way as guides for training purposes.

Two decision diagrams are presented here as examples: (1) *single weighing* (Fig. 4-2), and (2) *serial weighings* (Fig. 4-3). Both are based on the use of the two-line WHO growth chart, with an additional dotted "very low weight line" (−3 SD or 70%) beneath the main lines, and with six channels between the two main lines, marked by faintly dotted line and graded shading in the most culturally acceptable color. They can also be used, with appropriate modification, with the growth box systems employed in the Philippines (see Fig. 2.16) or developed by Essex and Gosling (1987) ("growth action records") (Fig. 2.17).

Single weighing. As emphasized several times, a single weighing is of very limited value and cannot be considered as growth monitoring. As mentioned earlier, it especially needs to be accompanied by an examination of the child and a history from the mother. A large child with the edema of kwashiorkor can be within the normal range; a low-weight child can be either wasted or stunted. The significance of a single low weight also needs to be judged in relation to subsequent weight gain as observed on the growth chart.

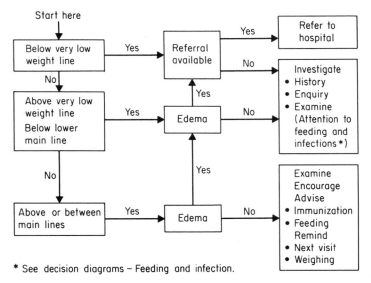

Figure 4-2   Decision diagram: single weighing.

Serial weighing. Unsatisfactory growth (inadequate weight gain, no weight gain or loss) (Fig. 4-3) needs investigation to try to identify dietary causes and infections that must be dealt with.

Most nonmalnourished children will show continuing increases in weight with growth curves between *and* paralleling (i.e., in the same general direction as) the two main lines.

Weight records between the main lower line and very low weight or emergency line need particular attention. Although such a record may be partially related to a low birth weight, a small mother, or genetic differences, the *probability* of abnormality is greater than with weight records higher on the graph. However, a chart showing a weight loss above the main lines also needs investigation. This can occur in a large and/or previously healthy child who is losing weight because of an inadequate diet, infections or, most usually, a mixture of several interacting causes.

IDENTIFICATION OF CAUSES AND ACTIONS

There are three primary causes of inadequate growth: *a deficient diet, infections,* and *poor child care.* These may be present singly or in combination.

Also, each primary cause can be due to a variety of secondary causes, which will vary in commonness from country to country and from family to family. In turn, there will be final causes or reasons, again with great variation from place to place. Some examples of the three levels of causes are given in Table

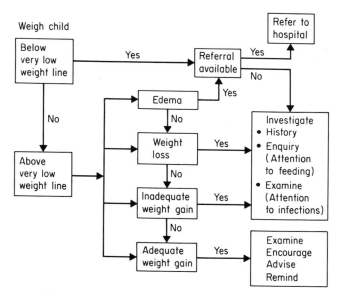

Figure 4-3 Decision diagram: serial weighings.

4-2. For training purposes, priorities need to be identified for particular communities, as will be discussed later.

Practical sources of information. In practice, the linking of growth monitoring to action depends on the simultaneous consideration of *four main sources of information* by the community health workers (Table 4-3), including the mother's history of the child, examination (mainly inspection), and knowledge of risk factors.

Sequence of activities during growth monitoring. Various sequences of activities can be carried out in different circumstances during growth monitoring in a community health workers' clinic or home visit or at collecting points. These may be undertaken by one community health worker during home visiting or at different "stations" in "lines of flow" in a village center with assistants, who may be volunteers.

In all these circumstances, other activities will also be undertaken as appropriate and convenient, including health and nutrition education (guidance and modification), immunization, advice on family planning, and so on.

Focusing on growth monitoring, the sequence of activities will be initiated by writing down some *general information* (such as date or month of attendance) followed by *weighing the child* (and writing down the weight) and *plotting the weight.* This is followed by an *inspection of the card,* including the child's growth line and the risk factors listed for the family, and *discussion*

Table 4-2 Some common primary and secondary causes of unsatisfactory growth

Main causes	Common secondary causes	Reasons
Deficient diet	Not enough breastfeeding	Mother dead or very ill
		Mother does not understand importance
		Mother unfamiliar with breastfeeding techniques (urban)
		Mother worried about baby's health or her figure
		Mother misled by advertisements
	Not enough family food or a poor mix of food going to the small child	Food not given frequently enough
		Food too dilute (insufficient *energy*)
		Food not of correct texture—not mashed enough
		Not enough peas and beans, food from animals, dark green leafy or orange vegetables in baby's diet
	Not enough food available to the family	Poverty, unemployment, broken family, single parent, no land for growing food
Infections	Communicable diseases	Diarrhea, acute respiratory infection (measles, whooping cough, etc.)
	Bad personal or food hygiene	Hygienic habits, such as handwashing and food storage (not keeping cooked food protected from flies)
	Bad community hygiene	Poor garbage or excreta disposal by family and community
Poor child care	Not enough time for looking after the baby well	Mother may go out to work, or too many household chores (fetching water or firewood)
	Not enough knowledge	Babysitter may be an older sister who does not understand her responsibilities, such as frequent feeding
	Not enough loving	Mother may be in need of company with whom to talk over her problems of child rearing
		Unwanted child (illegitimate; female babies in some cultures)
		Broken family (divorces, desertion, stepmother)
	An ill mother or caretaker	Tuberculosis, anemia, psychological problems

Table 4-3 Main sources of information needing consideration before taking action

Growth measurements (usually serial weighing)
Mother's history of the child
Diet
Infections
Examination of the child (mainly inspection)
General appearance
Some clinical signs[a]
Knowledge of risk factors for family and for the child

[a]Particularly edema, pale conjunctiva, dehydration or signs of infections, especially fever and the visible signs of a previous measles rash.

with the mother in which she gives a history of her child's symptoms (if any). After this, there will be an *examination of the child* for difficult to define, but often significant, "general appearance" and selected obvious clinical signs before finally deciding on what *action to take*. Of course, in some cases the mother may mention her child's symptoms and signs to start with, and at least partial examination may be undertaken earlier on. General inquiry into the current diet should be routine and results noted.

Focusing mainly on dietary deficiency and infections as causes of growth failure, two decision diagrams can be constructed for children with inadequate weight gain or weight loss in two age groups—young infants (0 to 6 months) (Fig. 4-4) and older infants and young children (6 months to 3 years) (Fig. 4-5).

Identifying causes and taking action. The actions most likely to be available in varying degrees to community health workers will be those concerned with feeding and infections. This is not to minimize the significance of family-social causes as risk factors. These also need investigation and as much action as feasible.

Dietary considerations. If a child's growth is found to be unsatisfactory by serial weighing, more detailed questioning concerning the diet is needed (Fig. 4-6), either at the time or soon after, when more time permits. The presence of infections also needs investigating by listening to the mother's history and hearing about her child's "presenting" or "current" main symptom, as discussed later.

Details of the questions asked will have to be related to the particular local pattern of infant feeding. If time permits (which it usually does not), models of domestic household measures and utensils (cups, spoons), and samples of uncooked foods (e.g., types of legume, oil) should be available. Uncommonly, even cooked, preserved samples of certain key items, such as staple preparations of different concentrations, may also be made available and can be very

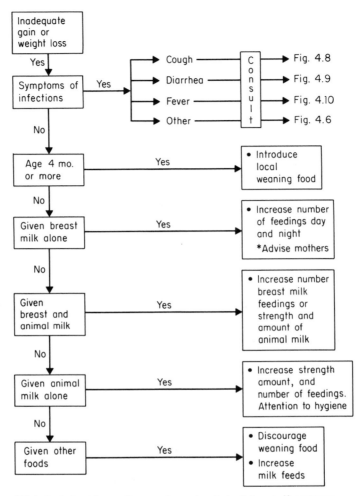

* If indicated advise mothers on improving their diet and, if necessary,
  issue supplements of iron, etc.

Figure 4-4   Management of inadequate weight gain or loss (infants 0 to 6 mo).

useful in nutrition education when discussing consistency. These may have specific local names (e.g., rice water, rice gruel, rice porridge). If an infant is being breastfed, it is most helpful to observe the mother and baby while nursing. This is especially so in urban circumstances, when very often young women have had no advice on the management of breastfeeding and may have had slight or no practical instruction from observation of successful nursing mothers. Minor changes in practical management, increased confidence, and more frequent sucking can often lead to rapid improvement in breastfeeding.

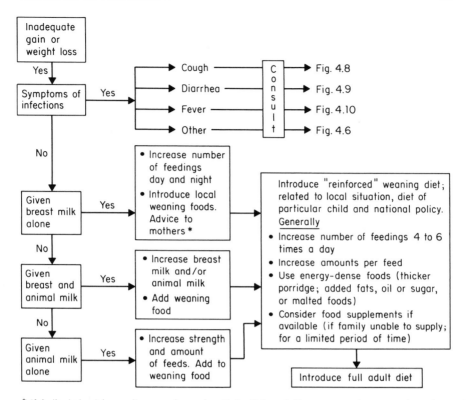

* If indicated advise mothers on improving their diet and, if necessary, issue supplements of iron, etc.

Figure 4-5   Management of inadequate weight gain or loss (6 mo to 3 yr).

Infections. Infections can play an important role in growth retardation because of poor appetite, increased nutritional needs (especially if fever occurs), and sometimes vomiting and diarrhea. Not infrequently, a further restriction of an already inadequate diet may be advised as an incorrect form of treatment, both by traditional and modern health workers.

Infections can sometimes be diagnosed by the community health workers from previous or present symptoms (e.g., whooping cough) or signs (e.g., Koplik's spots in the mouth and the characteristic rash in measles). Often, diagnosis and consequently treatment and management can only be suggested in an approximate way by the history of symptoms or signs reported by the mother or observed by the community health workers, and by the child's subsequent progress.

As one approach, a decision diagram based on the *main presenting symptom* reported by the mother may be useful (Fig. 4-7). The most common symptoms are cough, diarrhea, or fever. One problem with this approach is that it only

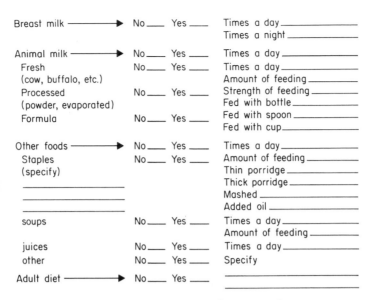

Figure 4-6   Approximate dietary inquiry.

includes the current main presenting symptom, which may have been different even a few days previously. Also, more than one symptom may be present. (Tentative "Decision Diagrams" for the three commonest main presenting symptoms just mentioned are given in Figs. 4-8, 4-9, and 4-10. These will need modification to suit local conditions in different countries or areas.)

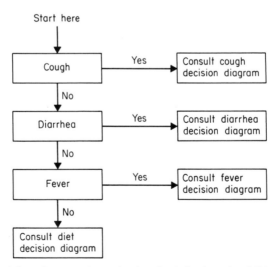

Figure 4-7   Decision diagram: investigation for infections in child with inadequate weight gain or weight loss (based on *main presenting* symptom reported by mother concerning child's history).

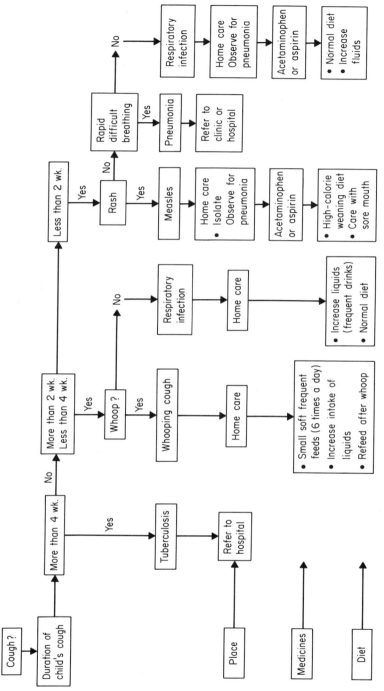

Figure 4-8 Main presenting symptom: cough.

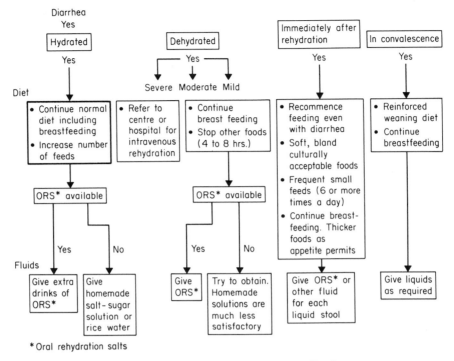

Figure 4-9 Main presenting symptom: diarrhea.

Family circumstances. In all societies, there are some families who are in need of extra or special care because of various biological, cultural, geographical, or economic circumstances that make them ''at risk'' or with a ''high risk'' of developing illness. This is particularly the case with malnutrition and infections in early childhood.

Special problem situations may be long term (chronic), such as extreme poverty, or may suddenly develop (acute), for example, the death of a parent. Locally serious problem situations need to be identified by the community health workers, as they require special attention. The identification of those at risk needs to be made in the course of home visiting, by questioning in the clinic, and by recording on the card. Often, the main risk factors are given in appropriate boxes on the child's growth chart or health card, sometimes listed as ''reasons for extra or special care.'' Such a specific listing is recommended, because otherwise they may be overlooked.

Such special care lists of risk factors can include examples at three levels.

1. *Community.* When a whole village or other large group is disadvantaged economically, culturally, geographically, seasonally, or various combinations of these.
2. *Family.* These may include the extremely poor, the landless, the low

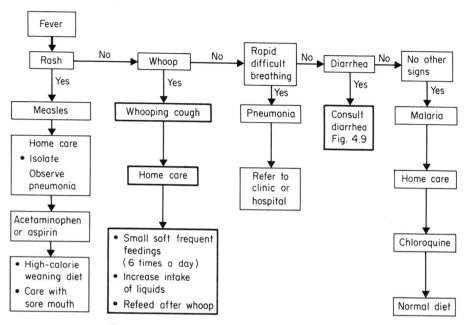

Figure 4-10 Main presenting symptom: fever.

caste or culturally less acceptable, or those with many, closely spaced children or with other previous children having been malnourished.

3. *Individual Child.* These will include the low birth weight, twins, the orphaned, and those who were bottle-fed.

Acute family disasters also may occur, creating emergency at-risk situations, from the death of a parent to an epidemic infection in the family livestock or a natural calamity, such as a drought or flood.

From a nutritional viewpoint, the most significant local risk factors need to be identified.[1] The degree of attention to be paid to them will depend on their perceived importance in causing malnutrition, how easy they are to recognize, and the feasibility of being able to help. Ideally, an epidemiological assessment of the relative significance of different risk factors can be made to assist community health workers. This is not often possible and, in any case, general judgments based on observation and feasibility of action always have to be made. Also, it can be assumed that the larger the number of at-risk factors present, the more children of such families need careful additional observation and supervision. This may include additional home visiting and special encouragement to attend for weighing more frequently, as well as special attention to protective actions, such as nutrition education, immunization, advice on family

1. From a more general perspective, these conditions may be health priorities for other reasons, including infectiousness and as direct causes of death.

planning, and methods of preparing oral rehydration solutions for use to prevent and manage dehydration in diarrhea.

SELECTION OF ACTIONS

The actions most likely to be available in varying degrees to community health workers will be those concerned with feeding and infections. This is not to minimize the significance of family-social causes leading to poor child care. These need investigation and as much action as feasible. Identification can best be made by reviewing the special care list on the child's record and by questioning the mother concerning recent events, which may have created new family-social stresses.

With regard to dietary deficiency and infections as causes of growth failure, two decision diagrams already mentioned (see Figs. 4-6 and 4-7) can be guides to appropriate actions.

Actions Available. These vary greatly with the child's condition and age, with local circumstances (as mentioned earlier), and with the training of the observer. *Much depends on having listened to the mother's main concerns.*

Essentially, actions can include different blends of the following.

- Praise and encourage (positive reinforcement).
- Advise and motivate (health education; some family-social problems).
- Routine activities appropriate for age (especially immunization).
- Specific realistic advice on improving the diet.[2]
- Supplementary food or nutrients *for defined periods* (including vitamin A capsules).
- Management of some infections (particularly oral rehydration for diarrhea).
- More frequent observation—by clinic attendance or home visiting according to circumstances.
- Referral to better-equipped health unit (e.g., health center or hospital), if feasible for parents as regards distance, means of transport, and time, and if services available are superior, or referral within the community, or arrangement for increased treatment at home.

Follow-up of Actions Taken. The success of advice given will have to be judged by observations at follow-up, including weighing. These should be at more frequent intervals than the regular weighings and at even closer intervals for young infants. Once again, details will have to vary with local circumstances, particularly the feasibility of mothers coming to a clinic or collecting point, or of the community health workers visiting homes. During such follow-up activities, in young infants, observation and weighing is indicated at least weekly.

2. Messages should be simple, culturally and economically feasible, clear, and relevant to the local feeding practices (Appendices E and F).

In older infants and young children, the weight should be recorded at least every 2 weeks.

If the child with previous growth failure is gaining in weight as indicated by a line moving upward, the special management initiated should be continued for a locally defined period of time. Usually this will be at least until the growth curve has continued upward for 4 weeks and preferably has returned to the channel believed to be appropriate for the particular child. However, at the same time, the child's history needs to be obtained from the mother to see if any major symptoms have persisted. These may indicate the need for referral despite an adequate weight gain. This can occur, for example, with a continuing fever.

If the child with previous growth failure is not gaining weight or continues to lose weight despite special management, detailed inquiry is needed from the mother concerning major symptoms and dietary intake. If the suggested increased dietary intake has not been followed (or cannot be, because of poverty), attempts should be made to insure that this is done, possibly by demonstration during home visits or by feeding at the clinic or other center, and/or the supply of supplementary foods. Again, selection depends on local circumstances.

If the major symptoms of infection continue with inadequate weight gain despite treatment available in the clinic and suggested increased dietary intake, referral is indicated, if feasible. If this is not possible, the community health workers must be encouraged to persist.

5

Alternative Growth Monitoring Systems

The best is the enemy of the good.
Voltaire (1764)

GENERAL

Many variables, including those summarized earlier, need to be considered in selecting a growth monitoring system that seems likely to work in a particular area. For various reasons given shortly, the ideal system often is not feasible. Instead, as suggested by Voltaire at the beginning of this chapter, overemphasis on unreachable complexity (''the best'') may so downgrade the idea of using the more limited activities that can be undertaken (''the good'') that the latter may not be considered. At the same time, programs need to be reviewed and changed as circumstances improve or deteriorate, with a better comprehensive system as the objective.

Such decisions need to be made following observation and overall analysis, including *decision-making workshops* and *focus-group discussions* (Manoff, 1985; Scrimshaw & Hurtado, 1987) (Appendix C) at different levels in particular countries or areas. Those involved should include *policymakers, technical experts, individuals carrying out practical growth monitoring (such as community health workers),* and *representatives of the community, especially mothers.* Often, a sequence of such decision-making workshops and discussions will need to be carried out at different levels of sophistication. These can culminate in joint meetings of all levels concerned with current WHO (1985) emphasis on *district health systems* as manageable units in primary health care. Some of these workshops could include district health teams, such as administrators and community representatives.

Usually six main considerations will influence decisions when designing a growth monitoring system.

1. *Financial.* Unappreciated cost of initial purchase of thousands of scales [1] (1988 UNICEF price for Salter scale—$30; market price about $35), to-

---

1. Bangladesh is stated to have about 68,000 villages. To supply one Salter scale for each village would cost approximately $2 million (UNICEF rate), or at least $2.4 million (general market rate).

gether with their repair and replacement, and of health cards (Home-Based Child's Record, (HBCR), especially if in attractive colors (as is desirable) and with a plastic protective envelope.

2. *Work-load.* Large numbers of mothers and children can overwhelm the community health workers and make weighing an inaccurate ritual, with no time available for explanation to mothers, and with inadequate opportunity for other activities, such as health education and immunization.

3. *Accessibility of Population.* Distance and isolation of dwellings and type of terrain[2] (e.g., mountainous, state of roads and rivers, etc.) influence the ability of mothers to attend clinics and of community health workers to make home visits; seasonal farming activities.

4. *Educational.* Problems with literacy and understanding of graphs, especially plotting and interpreting growth lines for appropriate action.

5. *Uninterrupted Availability of Clinic Supplies.* Medicines for minor illness, oral rehydration salts, educational aids for mothers, adequate (but not excessive) supplies of supplementary foods.

6. *Feasibility and Value of Referral.* Distance and difficulty and time for travel from clinic to health center and hospital (in relation to supervision and continuing training), and usefulness of doing so in relation to overcrowding and limited resources at the health center or hospital.

PRACTICAL SUGGESTIONS FOR DIFFERENT SYSTEMS

If a growth monitoring system is already in operation, it is suggested that the first approach should be to review it quietly, find any existing problems and, by appropriate modification or addition, try to overcome or circumvent them. Observation in many parts of the world has indicated the difficulty of completely changing a well-established system. This can lead to further confusion and irritation of the initiators of the system already in use.

If no system exists or if indicated by a preliminary investigation, alternative methods (or modifications) may have to be employed in growth monitoring systems, mainly using community health workers, in very differing circumstances in community clinics, in rally groups, or in the course of home visiting. The following suggestions are *not* comprehensive or inclusive, but are examples. Often, the difficulties or deficiencies mentioned here are multiple and combined. Not rarely, large numbers of children, inadequate funds, difficulties with graphing, and distant and inefficient supportive health services occur at the same time. Indeed, in some circumstances, any type of growth monitoring system will be impossible until at least minimal primary health care activities are introduced.

2. In Colombia, this has been recognized by the term *isochron* (literally, "equal time") to travel from home to clinic or vice versa (Pradilla, 1987). This concept helps to understand why a community health workers's ability to supervise a population of thousands of persons varies and cannot be laid down uniformly.

Situation A. Ideal
Characteristics

Enough well-trained, literate health workers, capable of regular, sequential monthly weighing and plotting on a graphic growth chart, preferably from birth onward, with funds available for sufficient numbers of scales and cards, with manageable numbers of young children from not-too-distant homes, with regular supplies available at community clinic or center [educational material for mothers, packets of oral rehydration salts (ORS), minor medicines, some supplementary foods], with follow-up, including transport to better-equipped health center and/or hospital practicable and with regular supportive supervision.[3]

Suggested System

Weigh all children as soon after birth as possible at agreed intervals (preferably monthly or as suggested by WHO)[4] *and* at any time that they attend for other reasons, such as immunization or illness. The weight can be plotted on a locally accepted chart emphasizing weight change as indicated by the slope of the growth line, with appropriate action feasible for inadequate weight gain and/or infections or by referral to available and appropriate better-equipped health services. Weighing should continue during the first 2 or 3 years of life, or longer, if circumstances permit.

Situation B. Very Large Numbers
Characteristics

As in Situation A, except for *very large numbers of young children* and no possibility of rapidly increasing numbers of community health workers (even including involving other health and nonhealth workers, such as agricultural extension agents, and possibly mothers and/or schoolchildren).

Suggested System

Consider restricting weighing (targeting) to a limited age range having greatest risk (e.g., 0 to 2 years), especially children from households known to be at risk because of individual or family circumstances, and/or those referred from the community following screening by arm tape measurement by community health workers during home visiting, or those found to be underweight in the course of measurement of village populations of young children at 3- to 6-month intervals at known collecting or rally points.[5]

---

3. Such characteristics are often assumed to be present. More often they are not in many less technically developed countries.

4. WHO (1986): one monthly—first year, two monthly—second year, three monthly—third year.

5. As in "Operation Timbang" in the Philippines (Nutrition Center of the Philippines, 1977).

Situation C. Inadequate Funds
Characteristics

As in Situation A, but *inadequate funds for sufficient number of scales.*

Suggested System

Pending development and widespread successful testing of low-cost, easily readable weighing devices such as the TALC scale (Morley, 1986), screen for thinness by serial measurements of arm circumference, either in the home or the village clinic, with the Zerfas insertion tape (p. 15) (Zerfas, 1975) or the "growth maintenance arm band" (Jelliffe & Jelliffe, 1989) (p. 36).

Situation D. Problems with Plotting
Characteristics

As in Situation A, with literate community health workers, but with *cultural problems with plotting weights on graph.*

Suggested System

Record weights in "weight boxes" as in the Philippine system (Griffiths, 1981) (p. 34) or the "growth action records" of Essex & Gosling (1987) (p. 35), or use a simplified system for weight plotting, as with the Bubble Chart (Griffiths, 1987) (p. 29) or the plotting device on the TALC scale (pp. 13 and 14) (Morley, 1986), or the Right-Way Weight Plotter (p. 33). However, all these methods need field testing in different circumstances.

Situation E. Widespread Illiteracy
Characteristics

As in Situation A, but *illiterate community health workers*

Suggested System

Use growth maintenance arm band (Jelliffe & Jelliffe, 1988b) (p. 36). Results from using a color-coded arm band would have to be recorded in colored boxes on the card (Zeitlin et al., 1982; Zeitlin, 1986; Jelliffe & Jelliffe, 1988b). The child's whole health card would have to be pictorial, using pretested, locally understandable pictures. This type of system needs to be tried in different circumstances, either alone or as part of a referral system where those children with low readings can be referred for weighing. This system needs replacing by serial weighing as soon as circumstances warrant it.

II
TRAINING FOR GROWTH MONITORING

We teach as we have been taught.
Jane Vella (1982)

As there is no universal method for growth monitoring, it follows that there can be no uniform content or system of training. Different systems have to be developed, depending on the many variations between communities and resources that have been discussed. Obviously, therefore, the content of training and the methods used cannot necessarily be replicated from one area or country to another, although general principles apply. Trial and adaptation are needed. It is especially important to avoid "pushing elaborate growth monitoring into a health system with (already existing) major weaknesses" (Gopalan, 1987) where there is no realistic chance of successful use on a wide scale and the danger of displacing other important activities.

6

Selecting A System

Two main questions have to be answered in each country or area: (1) *What system of growth monitoring is going to be used?* and (2) *What training program is needed?*

WHAT SYSTEM TO USE

As noted earlier (Chapter 3), great variations are to be found, especially in the size and distribution of the population (usually of children) to be included, the number and level of staff involved, funds available for the purchase, repair and replacement of equipment (such as weighing scales and clinic cards or HBCRs), the educational level of those expected to undertake growth monitoring, and the backup resources in terms of accessibility and level of health services for possible referral, supervision, and renewal of supplies.

A decision to try a particular growth monitoring system in a country or area needs to be based on information from different sources (Fig. 6-1). These will include knowledge of the health, nutrition, or other problems of the community and its resources and other characteristics: "community analysis" *and* result of decision-making workshops and focus-group discussions (Appendix C).

In some areas, a system of growth monitoring has already been established using, for example, a certain type of graph, such as one showing the Gómez weight lines (p. 24). It may be felt desirable to change this, [or some other components(s)] of whatever system is in place. As noted earlier, such actions must be approached with caution, as experience has shown great difficulty in effecting drastic changes in well-established practices. Sometimes it may be preferable to emphasize *better training,* possibly with some modifications. This will often have to include an understanding of what the lines used on the particular graph represent and the greater importance (and meaning) of the slope of the child's own growth line. Sometimes, change is essential—perhaps more commonly than believed—because of financial considerations, overwhelming numbers of children, cultural issues, and so forth (Chapter 3). In any case, a *single standardized, clearly understandable practical card* should be a national

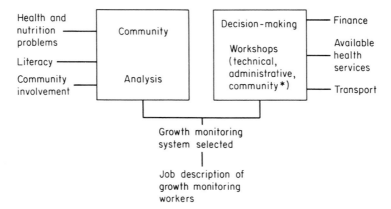

* Including focus discussion groups (Manoff, 1985; Scrimshaw & Hurtado, 1987) (Appendix C).

Figure 6-1   Selection of growth monitoring system; further details concerning variations are given elsewhere.

objective, if at all possible. In some countries, several very different weight charts may be used in different areas with much confusion. On the other hand, it may be necessary in a large country with varying circumstances to have two systems—one using serial weighing and the other screening or maintaining with color-coded arm bands for reasons outlined earlier (pp. 16, 36).

Methods of Selection

These will depend on knowledge of the different circumstances mentioned previously. If possible, selection should be made based on information obtained by community analysis concerning the variations made earlier (Table 6-1). In particular, *the opinions and views of parents, usually mothers, can be obtained by informal, friendly discussions,* by more organized focus-group interviews, or by combining results from questioning numbers of individuals. These methods are similar to those used in obtaining information from a particular segment of the population in commercial marketing surveys (Manoff, 1981).

In this way, it is possible to identify the main areas of cultural conflict (resistance points) and practical difficulties. At the same time, creative opportunities can be identified (Manoff, 1985). This will help in developing the most logical, practicable, and affordable growth monitoring system for the particular area, incorporating (rather than conflicting with) local cultural beliefs, such as mothers' reluctance to have their babies weighed in some parts of India. This will include agreeing on the *measurement* to be taken (usually weight), *method of recording* (usually plotting weights on a graph), *means of interpreting changes,* and *range of actions* available and how to select those most locally appropriate and possible. Such decisions will also obviously have to be based on many

Table 6-1   Some methods of selecting a local system of growth monitoring

Discussions with relevant health workers, trainers, administrators, and community members.

Written accounts.

Observation, preferably with descriptive research of the current system in operation and/or by watching activities at clinics, with an appropriate checklist.

Reviewing results in clinic and other available records regarding coverage and effectiveness

Interviews and focus-group discussions (Appendix C).

other matters. These particularly include the main workers to be responsible and their training; the site(s) where growth monitoring will take place (community center or clinic, home visits, collecting points); the equipment required for measurement; the equipment used for recording and for the management of infections; and, in appropriate circumstances, the food or nutrient supplements available or needed (e.g., vitamin A capsules). An estimate of overall cost will be a priority.

Details require much thought. These include, for example, what type of weighing scale can be afforded, what items to have on the card in addition to the growth chart (usually a weight graph), and how many years to cover (0 to 2 or 3 years or 0 to 5 years).

Only when an existing or new system has been agreed on can a logical national training program, based on principles given in this section, be devised. If at all possible, the system selected should then be tried out in a representative community or district health area, avoiding the frequent practice of using a highly atypical demonstration-teaching area with much larger than usual resources and a high-level of special attention. This is, of course, difficult to do, as the organizers understandably always have a close concern with the results. In many cases, modifications will often be found to be necessary, before wider replication can be considered—indeed, this is always a major problem. In some countries special modifications may be required in different cultural or linguistic areas, or if other factors differ greatly (e.g., educational level of community health workers). However, whenever possible one monitoring system with one type of graph (if serial weighing is used) should be the aim. The presence of different charts leads to unnecessary confusion in practice, in collection of comparable statistics and, most important, in large-scale training programs. In addition, consideration has to be given to incorporating training in growth monitoring into a curriculum covering the numerous other activities expected of the community health workers *and,* it must be reemphasized, into the practical training of supervisory health workers, including nurses, physicians, and nutritionists and, if possible, other village workers, such as agricultural extension workers, social workers, and schoolteachers.

Several systems have been suggested, and modifications in training related to them will be mentioned later (Chapter 7). These are only some alternatives given as examples. Realistic imagination needs to be given to modification or changes to suit local circumstances.

WHAT TRAINING PROGRAM IS NEEDED[1]

In whatever system is considered most locally useful, four basic questions need to be considered with regard to training: *Who? What? How? Where?*

Who to Train

The main cadre concerned with growth monitoring varies in different systems. In a limited number of areas, these will be physicians or, more commonly, nurses. However, most frequently, growth monitoring will be one of the responsibilities of a community health worker, whose educational background, length of training, and other duties vary greatly in different parts of the world (World Federation of Public Health Associations, 1984). This diversity is sometimes not recognized, and unwarranted generalizations can be made about the functions of the community health workers.

In a few exceptional circumstances, mothers themselves have been trained to weigh young children and chart their growth (Rohde et al., 1978). Elsewhere, in the child-to-child program, older schoolchildren have to be taught how to weigh and record results from younger children in the family (Aaron & Hawes, 1979). Training manuals also have been prepared for nonhealth-field workers, notably agricultural extension agents, to enable them to carry out this type of work (FAO, 1981).

Plainly, the cadre or cadres with main responsibility for growth monitoring in the country need priority in training, including those in government service and those working with nongovernmental organizations. However, at the same time, other members of the health team and the community also must be included in such activities. In fact, the chain of people with responsibility for understanding how to recognize growth failure and how to respond to it extends from the mother (and family) to the community health workers and his or her supervisor (often a nurse), to physicians at different levels of the health system, to public health administrators, and to political decision makers.

All members of the health team at all four WHO-designated levels (Table 6-2) need some training and/or orientation in growth monitoring, as well as other aspects of nutrition, especially of mothers and children. These include physicians, nurses, nutritionists, and dieticians. At present, any such educational coverage is mostly concerned with the temporary memorization of theoretical knowledge. Also, confusion can occur as a result of differences in factual detail in the training of different categories of health workers.

---

1. Numerous excellent texts are available on practical aspects of modern educational methodology, including Abbatt (1980), Guilbert (1982), and Guilbert et al. (1987). They emphasize "stimulating learning" rather than "force-fed teaching." They should be consulted and form part of the library of organizers' training programs.

Table 6-2 Four WHO-designated levels of workers involved in primary health care

Level 1	Level 2	Level 3	Level 4
Peripheral field workers	Supervisors and trainers of level 1 workers	Trainers of trainers, midlevel administrators, specialist and nonspecialist supervisors	Senior decision makers, high-level administrators, specialist and nonspecialist supervisors of level 3 workers

Most pediatric textbooks lack information on *practical skills* concerning growth monitoring. Often, medical students do not receive practical, hands-on training in weighing children or in filling in a growth chart; they get still less in how to interpret one or act on it. Physicians need this training if they are to give necessary support and scientific prestige to growth monitoring. Also, they are likely to be leaders of a health team, teachers, often ill-informed, of other health workers, and themselves directly responsible for the health care of children. In addition, an understanding of the economic, health, and scientific significance and practical issues involved needs to be included in the continuing education of senior administrators in a country's health service and political structure.

One aspect of modern trends in nursing training is toward greater involvement in primary health care (WHO, 1985). The development of the "Network"[2] for institutions concerned with health sciences is also a hopeful indicator that physicians and prestigious academic training establishments can become involved.

What Should Be Learned

Again, this depends on the system being used in the area, the personnel mainly responsible, and (often overlooked) the many other tasks they will be expected to carry out. These can sometimes be overwhelmingly, even unrealistically, extensive. Even nutrition-related tasks alone may be considerable (Table 6-3). Growth monitoring has to be integrated into primary health care services. Without this, it can become yet another vertical program.

The amount of theoretical background knowledge included or needed will vary greatly, for example, between a medical student and a trainee community health worker. Theoretical knowledge for any level of worker can be divided into (1) essential, (2) useful, and (3) interesting (but irrelevant for the practical tasks envisaged).

In all cases, the learning objectives must focus principally on an understanding of the rationale and aims of growth monitoring and then on the practical

2. Network of Community-Oriented Educational Institutions for Health Services, Secretariat, University of Maastricht, The Netherlands.

Table 6-3 Learning objectives for training in nutrition for community
health workers

Understand the commoner causes of unsatisfactory growth in the local community (feeding practices, infections, poor child care).

Understand the concept of growth and the factors that promote or retard normal growth.

Weigh an infant or child accurately.

Record the weight on the growth chart used in the service.

Insert correctly any other information required in the chart.

Assess normal growth on a growth chart.

Assess deviations from normal growth on a growth chart.

Interpret deviations in terms of health status.

Translate the information on the growth chart into appropriate advice and action.

Recognize the need for, and make decisions regarding, the referral of patients to a higher level of the health system.

Use the growth chart as an integral part of the health care system.

Recognize how to motivate and involve mothers in appreciating the value of growth monitoring.

Explain to mothers the use and significance of the growth chart.

Modified from WHO, 1986b.

tasks and detailed skills needed for the five activities used in the particular local system—that is: *motivating* → *measuring* (usually weighing) → *recording* (usually plotting on a weight chart) → *interpreting* → *taking action*.

Details need defining by task analysis in the particular situation, that is, related to the educational level and general situation of the worker and to the instruments and resources available for the growth monitoring system used. By this means, decisions concerning the detailed practical skills needed can be made and a curriculum designed showing learning objectives, teaching methods, ways trainees are assessed, and timetables.

How to Train

Training at all levels should be concerned principally with enabling students to learn the skills needed for the tasks required of the particular type of worker in the growth monitoring system being used. Learning should be active—*combining* describing and demonstration by the trainer with doing (practice) (Fig. 6-2). Involvement of students in practical work should be the main method used (Table 6-4), including problem solving, group discussion, and role playing. Evaluation—that is, testing the students' understanding and practical performance—should be included at all stages, as will be outlined in Chapter 7.

Practical learning should progress, when possible, from *initial training* (moving from simulation to reality), to *in-service training* (apprenticeship or on-the-job

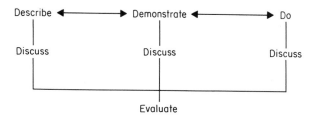

Figure 6-2 Practical combined sequence in training.

experience, assisting in fieldwork), to actual *fieldwork* (with follow-up by *supportive* supervision and intermittent refresher courses, without which they feel neglected and unimportant, and their knowledge becomes out of date). Supportive supervision includes praise for work well done, friendly suggestions concerning inadequacies, review of supplies and equipment, satisfactoriness of the referral system and, above all, giving prestige to the community health workers by working with him or her and making it clear that the results are appreciated and are producing benefit.

Where to Train

Again, this will vary with the cadre concerned. For medical and nursing students, growth monitoring needs to be included in their curriculum, both in theory *and in practice*. It also should be a part of the other aspects of clinical work considered to be scientific and prestigious. These include endocrinology and the evaluation of improvement or deterioration of patients in hospital.

Realistic practical training should take place as much as possible in sites with similar conditions to the actual work places (Table 6-5). This applies not only

Table 6-4 Tasks presented as modules to be covered in nutrition training for community health workers

Module 1. Getting to know the community and its needs.

Module 2. Measuring and monitoring the growth and nutrition of children.

Module 3. Promotion of breastfeeding.

Module 4. Nutritional advice on the feeding of infants and young children.

Module 5. Nutritional care of mothers.

Module 6. Identification, management, and prevention of common nutritional deficiencies.

Module 7. Nutritional care during diarrhea and other common infections.

Module 8. Conveying nutrition messages to the community.

Module 9. Solving nutritional problems in the community.

From WHO, 1986b.

Table 6-5 Advantages of community location for training

Training content and methods can be easily adapted to local circumstances.

It facilitates attendance by women and others with ongoing community responsibilities.

Trainees can more easily practice fieldwork skills.

Local residents can observe and perhaps participate in the course.

Communities can help defray trainee expenses.

It facilitates participation by supervisors who will work with health workers after training.

Trainees may be able to walk to training sites.

Trainers at a central institution are unlikely to have posttraining contact with health workers.

Trainers at a central institution are unlikely to be knowledgeable about local circumstances and the health worker's work environment.

It encourages use of appropriate technology, such as locally made audiovisual aids, and basic rather than sophisticated medical equipment.

From World Federation of Public Health Associations, 1983a.

to community health workers, but also to medical and nursing students. The latter need exposure and experience of this type, both as part of their general professional education and because they need to appreciate the significance and difficulties of the work of other team members, especially community health workers, for whom they will often be the trainers.

7

Designing Training

Once a growth monitoring system has been decided on, realistic, workable *job descriptions* need to be laid down for the individuals who will be involved and a *training program* designed. In many circumstances, most monitoring will be by community health workers, often with little formal education, working under very difficult conditions, and with limited resources.

The logical design of training needs to be considered in two steps (modified from Abbatt, 1980): (1) *definition of learning objectives—tasks,*[1] *subtasks,* and *KSA (Knowledge-Skills-Attitudes)* needed, including specific consideration of three types of skills: *manual* (psychomotor—skilled use of hands), *mental* (reasoning, thinking, decision making), and *communication* (explaining, persuading) (Fig. 7-1); and (2) *practical considerations* to cover these learning objectives, including *lesson plans, teaching methods* (and *aids*), *timetable,* and *evaluation* (Fig. 7-2).

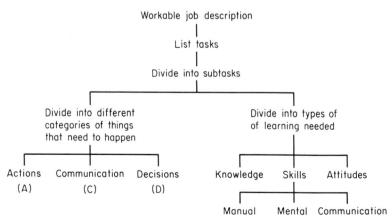

Figure 7-1 Learning objectives for growth monitoring workers (based on Abbatt, 1980).

1. A task is a main, identifiable job or piece of work.

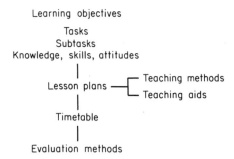

Figure 7-2   Curriculum design (modified from Abbatt, 1980).

LEARNING OBJECTIVES

Examples of learning objectives for health workers using growth charts are given in Table 7-1.

All aspects of the five-part sequence, previously noted as employed in growth monitoring—*motivating, measuring, recording, interpreting* and *taking action* (Fig. 1-1)—are currently being critically reappraised in different parts of the world. Indeed, a wide review of all steps in this process in required (as in this book), because the later stages of the sequence—decisions and actions—are dependent on the earlier ones.

Although not often appreciated, an essential element in recruitment, training and continuity is that of incentives for the community health worker. We cannot go into this vital and controversial issue here. Apart from the availability of more obvious immediate rewards (financial incentives and privileges), the motivation of community health workers must include other considerations, such as pride, prestige, compassion, and possible opportunities for advancement.

Potential difficulties can occur at all stages, including weighing and plotting. However, serious problems often arise with interpretation and decision making that lead to appropriate actions being taken.

Two main priorities seem to exist.

1. Adapting methods and equipment used for growth monitoring to the very variable local circumstances and resources in different parts of the world (community or situation analysis) based on advice and discussion with all concerned, especially with local workers and members of the community, particularly mothers (to enable the ''user's view'' to be given priority).
2. Devising practical effective training suitable for the educational level and culture of workers in a particular area, based on the equipment and methods already employed in that area (or making needed changes), and with special emphasis on interpreting results for decision making and action.

The need for devising training, which is both adjusted to local needs and effective, is the main theme of this book. However, this cannot be undertaken

Table 7-1 Suggested task analysis form: Subtasks in task of plotting weight on graphic growth chart by community health worker

Category of worker: Community health worker
Task: Recording (plotting) weight on growth chart

Subtasks Actions (A) Decisions (D) Communications (C)	Knowledge	Skills	Attitudes
1. Obtain knowledge of weight (written or verbal direct from scale)[a]	Ability to read scale used	Literacy	
2. Check months recorded correctly	Understand calendar months	Read months	
3. Identify present month[b] 4. Identify present weight 5. Plot weight with dot	Understand structure of graph	Ability to plot weight (using chart lines or recent innovations, such as the TALC chart (Annex 1) or the Bubble Chart (Annex 3) or the Right-Way Weight Plotter (Annex 9)	Care and accuracy
6. Judge recent weight change	Recognize meaning of different slopes	Join recent dots with a line (growth line)	

[a] Depends on procedure in clinic and whether one person weighs and plots, or whether two are responsible.
[b] Ability to plot to approximately the right period in the month, varies with the size of the space in the chart between months and the understanding of the community health worker.

logically and with greatest influence without recognizing the many alternatives and variables in methods and circumstances mentioned earlier.

TASK ANALYSIS

This type of detailed analysis is often difficult for professionals trained in an orthodox manner to appreciate or conceptualize. Their own education may have emphasized mainly factual knowledge, with skills and attitudes often learned informally and in an unplanned way as part of observation and apprenticeship. For medical students, for example, the latter would include ward rounds, followed by supervised experience as interns/house physicians.

Sometimes this difference between knowledge-based and competency-based training (Table 7-2) can be better understood by highly trained health professionals if examples are considered from manuals on how to repair a car or operate a videotape recorder.

Table 7-2 Comparison of knowledge-based and competency-based training

Knowledge-based training	Competency-based training[a]
Organization of content around academic topics such as antomy, physiology, and disease vectors	Organization of content around specific functions, such as identification and treatment of diarrhea, motivation of community leaders, etc.
Emphasis on knowledge	Emphasis on attitudes and skills
Limited skill practice	Extensive skill practice
Use of competitive exams, mainly designed to evaluate rather than assist students	Use of noncompetitive exams to verify competencies and help students and trainers identify weak areas
Attitude that students must adapt to the teaching method	Attitude that teaching method must be adapted to the student
Use of scaled-down nursing or other educational curricula	Use of task analysis to base curricula on specific community health worker functions
Separation of theory and practice	Close conjunction between theory and practice, preferably taught concurrently

From WHO, 1986b.
[a]Task-oriented training (Abbatt, 1980; Guilbert, 1982).

Such analyses are time consuming. It often seems easier to scale down or simplify the knowledge previously received by the would-be trainers. For some professionals, including physicians, the whole process may seem obvious, ''unacademic,'' boringly trivial, and beneath their attention. This is not so—competency-based practical training is needed in any field, from astronauts to neurosurgeons. It is certainly very much required for the training of community health workers in growth monitoring. They may have particular additional difficulties with limited literacy, unfamiliarity with straight lines, the decimal system or graphs, and the other local cultural problems and differences, as noted earlier. *Lack of realization of the need for this type of educational approach seems to be one of the more remediable reasons for inadequate or inappropriate training and for consequent poor performance.* It can certainly be one important reason for current dissatisfaction regarding growth monitoring in some parts of the world.

The following examples are given to illustrate the task-related approach using the most commonly described system of growth monitoring (System A: Ideal) (p. 60).

Tasks and Subtasks

As noted several times, growth monitoring in the conventionally described manner comprises five main tasks: *motivating, weighing, recording* (including filling out other sections of the card as well as plotting the weight), *interpreting,* and *taking joint action* by the mother and the community health workers. The last four tasks are often carried out at a village center established by a community health worker, but they can be undertaken during home visits or at village collecting points, depending on the details of the system employed.

Task 1   Weighing

The subtasks needed will vary with the situation, including, for example, the type of scale used, where the weighing is done, the way in which the clinic (or other weighing site) is organized, and the number of workers involved in the process from measurement to recording to interpreting to taking action.

Subtasks have to be given in *considerable detail*—much more so than is usually appreciated. For instance, the listing concerning "weighing a baby in an MCH clinic" (Abbatt, 1980) (Table 7-3) is insufficient for community health workers training. In this, the whole process is presented as a single task. It should be regarded as at least four tasks: weighing (including testing and taring the scale), recording, interpreting, and taking action. Each task then needs breaking down into subtasks.

Table 7-3   General task analysis form (Abbatt, 1980)

Category of worker: Nursing orderly
Task: Weighing a baby in MCH clinic (Abbatt, 1980)

Subtasks 　Actions　　　　(A) 　Decisions　　　(D) 　Communications (C)	Knowledge	Skills	Attitudes
1. Ask mothers to dress babies in weighing trousers　(C)		Ability to explain why; dress babies in weighing trousers	Friendliness to mothers
2. Place baby on scale　(A)		Reading scales; handling babies	Accuracy
3. Help mother take off weighing trousers; examine baby　(A)		Recognition of signs of malnutrition	Thoroughness
4. Record weight on growth chart　(A)		Plotting points on graph	Accuracy
5. Decide whether to comment to mother or report to more senior staff　(D)	When report is necessary normal weights for babies of various ages		
6. Report or comment as necessary　(C)	What comments or reports to make	Report writing; communicating to mothers	Concern for baby's health; respect for mother

Table 7-4   Task analysis form: using a Salter scale or a local beam balance
(following Abbatt system)

Category of worker: Community health worker
Task: Weighing young child in rural primary health clinic

Subtasks
  Actions   (A)
  Decisions   (D)
  Communications   (C)
	Knowledge	Skills	Attitudes

At beginning of session			
1. Suspend scales securely at eye level (A)	Sites for suspension	Suspension system of scales used	Practicality
2. Return scale reading to zero ("tare") (A)	Mechanism for returning to zero	Know how to use mechanism	Accuracy
3. Test accuracy of scales (A)	Variation in scales with use and time	Know how to make and use test weights	Accuracy
For each child			
4. Ask mother to undress child (C)[a]		Assist mother	Courtesy; friendliness
5. Place child in weighing trousers (or) sling (C, A)	Avoid mother holding child or feet touching ground	Handling children	Reassurance
6. Note or read out weight (A)		Ability to read scales	Accuracy
7. Write down weight reading in figures (self or assistant) (A)		Literacy	Accuracy
8. Assist mother to remove child (C, A)		Handling children	Gentleness; comforting
9. Record weight (graph; box) (A)[b]	Ability to understand record system used		Accuracy

[a]Completeness of undressing depends on weather and culture (mother's attitudes).
[b]Recording of weight can best be considered as a separate task.

Some of the subtasks that need to be *D*escribed, *D*emonstrated and *D*one in such a simple-seeming task as weighing are given in Table 7-4, together with "things that need to happen" (actions, decisions, communications) and knowledge, skills, and attitudes (Abbatt, 1980). Some of these are illustrated in Fig. 7-3 (Kigondu, 1986).

In fact, the task of weighing itself has to be preceded by two others. The first is convincing and motivating mothers to bring their babies for weighing.

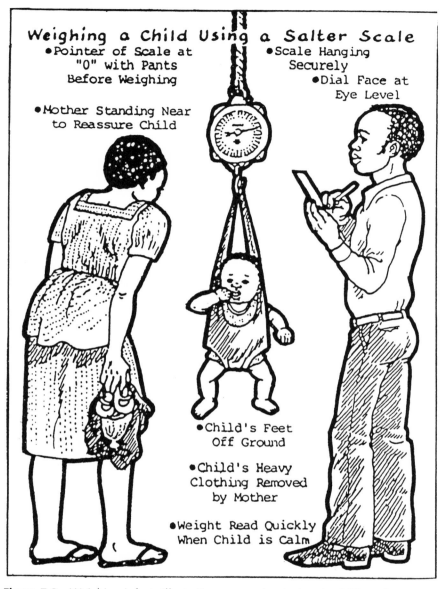

Weighing a Child Using a Salter Scale
- Pointer of Scale at "0" with Pants Before Weighing
- Scale Hanging Securely
- Dial Face at Eye Level
- Mother Standing Near to Reassure Child
- Child's Feet Off Ground
- Child's Heavy Clothing Removed by Mother
- Weight Read Quickly When Child is Calm

Figure 7-3 Weighing infant: illustrating some subtasks involved (Kigondu, 1986). (Note: recorder should be *directly facing* the dial of the scale.)

This can be difficult in some cultures, such as in some areas of India, where weighing may be considered dangerous (e.g., risk of babies being exposed to bewitchment from the ''evil eye,'' etc.), or demeaning, being similar to weighing food at a market (Gopalan & Chatterjee, 1985; Abel, 1986).

The second task prior to weighing is the correct filling out (or checking) of other items on the card, including the month of the present attendance in the calendar boxes on the card.

Task 2   Recording

Recording may be on a weight graph (chart) or using a weight box system (Fig. 2-16 and 2-17), or a color-coded bar graph (Fig. 2-18).

Plotting on a weight graph often can be difficult because graphs are culturally foreign to those with limited formal modern mathematical education in many communities. The recently introduced TALC scale (p. (Fig. 2-2) or the Bubble Chart (Fig. 2-13) are currently being tested and may help in simplifying plotting. In the meantime, the task of weight plotting should be broken down into subtasks (Table 7-1), with the possible assistance of the "Right-Way Weight Plotter" (Fig. 2-15).

In the Philippines, it has been suggested that the weight box system is more easily followed by community health workers and mothers.

Task 3   Interpreting

Interpreting is usually difficult as it involves two subtopics; assessing growth and judging the main causes.

Assessing Growth. Rather than using the type of analysis used for weighing and recording, the following decision sequence can be used.

1. Position of the most recent weight dot on the chart (for first weighing or after prolonged failure to attend).
2. *Examination of the slope of the growth line,* made by joining the last two or preferably three weight dots and recognition of satisfactory growth versus unsatisfactory growth (including no gain, inadequate gain, or weight loss) (Chapter 3).
3. Decision on *general* actions to be taken, considering different alternatives, preferably guided by appropriate decision diagrams (Figs. 4-6 to 4-10) according to categorization of the growth line (see point 2).

Task 4   Deciding on Action

The action or actions to be taken will depend very much on local circumstances, as indicated earlier. They will also be influenced by three other sources of information ("decision support systems") (Essex & Gosling, 1987), as well as the weight changes. These are (1) the mother's history of the child (diet, infections), (2) examination of the child (general appearance and some obvious clinical signs), and (3) a knowledge of the risk factors for the family and for the particular child (Chapter 4).

To decide on actions with regard to feeding, decision diagrams can be constructed for young infants (0 to 6 months) (Fig. 4-4) and for older infants and young children (Fig. 4-5), together with consideration of some details of feeding (Fig. 4-6).

If results suggest that an infection may be most significant, a decision diagram of the three main symptoms can be used (Fig. 4-7). In turn, these may lead to a review of a decision diagram for the particular symptom (Fig. 4-8, 4-9, and 4-10).

All such decision diagrams or lists (''management options'') (Essex & Gosling, 1987) need to be devised for the particular locality.

The actions available must be simplified, specific and, as far as possible, standardized. For example, the term ''action package'' has been suggested (Essex & Gosling, 1987) for the three elements needed for children who are growing well—''praise, encourage, routine activities'' (such as immunization appropriate for age). In Indonesia, standardized messages have been devised concerning dietary advice for different common situations encountered there (Sukmanah, 1987) (Appendix F).

8
Practical Considerations

CURRICULUM DESIGN

The curriculum will need to be designed to cover the tasks that will be required for the individual's work, as given in his or her job description.

Topics, sometimes termed modules, to be covered will include the following.

- *Relationship between growth and health.*
- *Causes of growth failure:* diet, infections, poor child care.
- *Concept of risk factors.*
- *Layout of locally used card* and how to fill out name, social details, month of birth and current date, other information needing to be filled in, and meaning of messages and information.
- *Weighing scale:* appearance, meaning of markings on scale, taring (returning zero), testing (with appropriate weights).
- *Weighing:* writing down weight (guided by task analysis).
- *Plotting:* on graph or box (guided by task analysis) (Chapter 2).
- *Interpreting:* slope of growth lines and position on graph (see Chapter 4).
- *Selecting actions:* (Chapter 4).
- *Preparing teaching material* (Abbatt, 1980; Barclay et al., 1982).

LESSON PLANS

These need to be developed for each topic (module). They can be planned in detail, but always must remain flexible to allow as much opportunity as possible for discussion and feedback from students. They must include (1) the task of the trainer, (2) the teaching materials and equipment used, (3) the proposed activity by the trainer, (4) the proposed activity by the students, and (5) the trainer-student interaction. Appropriate sequences need to be considered for different topics.

TEACHING METHODS

Training should be informal, with as much active involvement of the students as possible, especially in practical work, including problem solving. This can

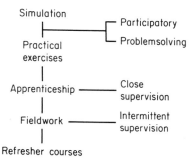

Figure 8-1   Progression of training: with involvement of mothers at all stages.

be helped by simple devices such as sitting in a circle and encouraging non-threatening discussion. The latter may be more difficult in some cultures where women are conceived as passive and thus unlikely to question the teacher or enter into discussion.

The role of teachers should be as friendly helpers and communicators, not as didactic, authoritarian superiors. They are trying to assist students to acquire specific skills ("facilitators"), but also to learn themselves. They should represent role models, as indicated by body language and avoidance of "talking down," both in vocabulary and methods.

Common practices of giving general didactic information and blanket answers should be avoided (Tremlett, 1985). Specific basic facts and skills need to be acquired by lessons that should also try to sustain interest and entertain. Lessons should contain an appropriate blend of description, demonstration, and discussion. They should include built-in nonalarming, "quiet," informal evaluation of the students' understanding, progress, and practical ability, as judged by pre-and posttesting.

Demonstrations of practical skills by teachers need to be arranged carefully. They must be visible to the class and explained at the same time by whoever is carrying them out, whether teacher, student, or both together.

Training should move from theory to practice (Fig. 8-1): *simulation* to *practical exercises* (including *problem solving*) to *closely supervised apprenticeship* to *fieldwork* (with *intermittent supervision*). However, these should not be considered separate stages. They can be blended in various ways appropriate to the particular situation.

TIME AND LOCATION

The length and continuity of *initial training* will have to be decided depending on local circumstances and will need to be worked out, as will a timetable. Often, training may be initiated by a "short" course, preferably held and organized near the students' field of work or in similar conditions. The length of such a course can only be decided on after a logical and detailed curriculum has been defined and integration with training for other tasks is planned. This needs to be modified subsequently, as shown by experience with its use and by evaluation of its effectiveness as indicated by the subsequent performance of trainees. However, other practical considerations will affect the length of a course, including the cost and the periods of time students can be away from home, especially women in some cultures.

The risk of overloading students' minds with too many facts in too short a time also needs consideration. Other alternatives include a very brief introductory course, followed by sessions or short blocks of training.

CONTINUING TRAINING

This is a lifelong process—at all levels. For the community health workers in particular, this needs to be undertaken, mainly informally during visits by the worker's supervisor and by occasional short refresher courses. Without these, enthusiasm and interest almost inevitably decline, and a feeling of unimportance and isolation develops.

TEACHING–LEARNING AIDS

These can be divided into (1) *procedures,* and (2) *audiovisual (AV) devices.* They may be classified in several ways. Here we divide them by cost and complexity, because these relate to the likelihood of their availability and understandability. It must be emphasized that teaching aids mentioned are intended to try to help in the use of the customary monitoring equipment—usually weighing scales and growth charts. Reality and practice should be the main AV aids, with as much involvement of, and interaction with, mothers and their children.

Procedures

These range from *stimulating (but friendly) questioning* to more complex procedures. These include *storytelling* (CONTACT, 1987).[1] They can have a clearcut message or may be open ended, where the group is left with the question, "What would you do?" Sometimes, this can be made less worryisome for more shy individuals, especially women in some cultures, by using some method to indicate response by the whole group.

In some circumstances, mothers' classes may be given as part of the training. In any case, the involvement of experienced mothers in these exercises can be helpful, if the community health worker does not feel she is losing status by doing so.

1. Unstructured stories are available from CONTACT, Christian Medical Commission, World Council of Churches, 150 Route de Ferney, Geneva, Switzerland.

Table 8-1   Projects or exercises for students—depending on level of education

1. Making your own local events calendar
2. Making and interpreting a growth chart
3. Practicing weighing a baby and filling in a growth chart
4. Role playing about filling in a growth chart for a new baby
5. Interpreting growth charts
6. Identifying mistakes on growth charts
7. Field evaluation of use of growth charts

An additional stimulus to thinking and decision making can be provided by various *games* (including picture cards) and *projects and exercises* undertaken by students (Table 8-1).

Another technique is the *focus group discussion* (Appendix C), in which class members respond and interact to a real or devised situation and/or guided questions. The method is a very helpful way of involving students and overcoming shyness, leading to interaction and discussion and, what is more, teaching the teacher. More experienced, convinced mothers particularly need to be included.

More practical procedures include the *simulated use of actual equipment*. Examples of this include weighing procedures with model baby dolls (including testing scales and taring to zero), some techniques to increase the weight, such as the "bucket system"[2]; moving to weighing actual young children, preferably with markedly differing weights. At more advanced stages, such exercises would include plotting, interpreting and deciding on appropriate action(s) in consultation with mothers, using actual charts or enlarged versions, or flannel graphs.

A common mistake is to use a graph showing weight changes over many months. This is useful for the experienced, but blurs the main message. The most instructive growth lines are those focusing on weight changes over a 2- to 3-month period, as this needs to be their main concern in practice.

A most effective and often entertaining procedure, requiring considerable care in planning, is *role playing*. Most students enjoy this type of activity. They soon come to recognize some of the issues, attitudes, and problems of both mothers and fellow workers, especially if they change roles. A less direct form of role playing can be by the use of home made *puppets*.

In training in growth monitoring, problems, concerns, or situations that could be considered for role-playing sessions include (1) the apprehensive new mother of the child, (2) the father objecting to wife and child's attendance, especially for weighing, (3) the detection of unsatisfactory growth and possible cause, and (4) effects of unexpected problems (risk factors) on a family, especially on the growth of their young children.

2. Using a model doll weighed in a bucket, into which water can be poured to increase the weight (Morley, 1986).

AV Aids

Audiovisual (AV) aids differ greatly in cost and complexity (Table 8-2). Their use in the various procedures just summarized, and in the progress from simulation to actual work, will also differ with many local circumstances. However, all may play a part in different circumstances, depending on funds, level of literacy, and so on. In particular, their message(s) should be simple, clear,

Table 8-2 Teaching-learning audiovisual aids: A selection

1. *Low-cost aids*		
Visual aids		

Live examples
  (well, grown child; healthy
  vs. sick animal; spindly vs.
  normal carrot)		

Pictures
  (printed or homemade drawings
  or photographs)
	Poster size
	Large or small cards;
	flip charts
		Single: one message
		Comparative: well-nourished
		child vs. malnourished child
		Serial: storytelling (? with message on back or elsewhere as guide for teacher)

Games		
Models	Cardboard Flannel	*Enlarged* dial To help of scales reading and *Enlarged* flannel recording graph of growth results chart (showing weights from birth)
Written aids		
Checklists of activities		Initial visit Subsequent visits
Counseling cards		Picture on front with explanation and questions on reverse
Mimeographed workbooks (or sheets)		Checklist of tasks (in sequence) Detailed mainly pictorial instructions on tasks
2. *More expensive aids*		
Books		Workbooks Reference/guidance manuals Picture books (comic books/photonovellas)
Mechanical equipment (needing electricity)		Slides[a] Filmstrips Films Videocassettes Interactive videodiscs

[a]One example is the slide set *Charting a Child's Growth*, available from TALC, P.O. Box 49, St. Albans, Herts., All-4AX, UK.

Table 8-3 Content of training manual used in Kenya

Reasons for the new child health card.

How to fill in the front of the card.

How to record information on immunizations.

How to use the child health card to improve the growth and nutrition of children.

The growth chart.

Remember to fill in the birth date of the child.

How to weigh a child accurately with a hanging scale.

Entering the weight on the growth chart.

How to interpret the growth line.

The meaning of the printed lines on the growth chart.

What mothers should know about the chart.

Other information that should be entered on the chart.

How often a child should be weighed.

How to make sure that the scale is working properly.

How information from the charts can be used to help the community improve health and nutrition.

How to find the child's age.

From Nutrition Division, Ministry of Health/UNICEF.

uncluttered, understandable, culturally appropriate, and within the "pictorial literacy" of the audience. Pretesting is essential, followed by modification, if needed.

The mechanical aids mentioned are costly to varying degrees. When possible, they also need to be carefully prepared with assistance from artists and communication experts, and particularly need to be pretested on intended audiences in the particular culture, since some Western, well-established communication conventions are not necessarily easily understood. An example is the "fade-out, fade-in" technique used in movies—in which it is recognized that time has passed between the two scenes.

LEARNING PACKAGES

These packages will vary, depending on circumstances and the level of training under consideration.[3] All learning packages will have to be based on the availability of the growth monitoring equipment used locally. They will usually comprise mainly "how-to" *manuals* (Table 8-3) for (1) trainers (with greater

1. For example, the Nutritional Division, Ministry of Health, Nairobi, Kenya (with UNICEF assistance) has two small booklets plus slide sets on growth promotion. One is entitled, "Using the Kenya Child Growth Chart," and the other, "Growth Monitoring Case Studies." Both are intended mainly for trainers of community health workers.

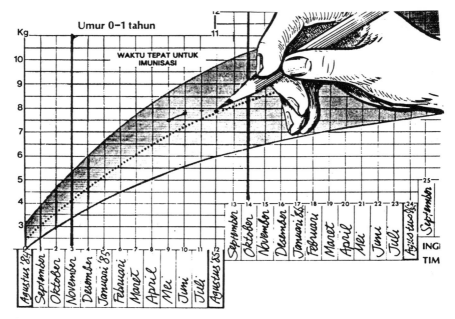

Figure 8-2   Clear, simple illustration of plotting weight (Indonesia) (UPGK, 1985).

detail and explanation), and (2) trainees [after training, often largely pictorial (Fig. 8-2), showing tasks broken down into subtasks, etc.], to be used for teaching mothers, as instruction guidebooks for use in practice, and as *teaching-learning aids* (such as those indicated earlier). In addition, small libraries and other equipment will be invaluable for trainers and trainees, but at different levels of complexity and sophistication.

III
EVALUATION

Evaluation should be planned prior to modification or innovation. If funds permit, this can be carried out scientifically by experts in this field, with technical guidance from those with in-depth knowledge of the issues involved in all aspects of growth monitoring in the particular area. Evaluation should never be undertaken by experts with no firsthand knowledge of local reality. In all cases, a period of field involvement—or at least observation—is absolutely mandatory.

Such a process should include assessment of (1) the growth monitoring system under trial, and (2) the effectiveness of the training program as regards the trainees, the teachers, and the community.

At its simplest, it is important to obtain some data on numerical coverage and information on acceptability and usefulness from community health workers *and* from mothers. This will not give exact results, but it is useful and can be obtained fairly easily by observation, discussion, and review of numbers of children whose growth has been monitored.

Indeed, as noted by Feuerstein (1986), many methods for evaluating community health projects are "too complex, too costly or not appropriate to the real conditions." In addition to the collection of detailed facts and figures through surveys, she advises "partnership in evaluation" among the community, the health workers, and the evaluator.

By looking carefully at what is *actually* happening to appreciate achievements, weaknesses, and realities, for such "participatory evaluation" Feuerstein (1986) recommends: (1) *a review of records with mothers,* (2) *case studies*—observation of one or two training centers and *monitoring* growth monitoring clinics, and (3) *community meetings and discussions.*

9

Growth Monitoring System

If a new or a modified system is introduced, the study design shown in Fig. 9-1 should be used, if feasible. If a system is already in operation, results may be compared from an ''intervention area'' with a carefully selected similar control area of the country in which the system is not present.

In such comparisons, statistical advice on sampling is essential and the areas selected must avoid the common faults of ''pilot projects'' or ''demonstration areas.'' These have unrealistic levels of funding, staffing, and personal support from enthusiastic initiators of the whole activity. Those evaluating should be thoroughly aware of the local situation but, if at all possible, should not be members of the team involved in making the changes being evaluated. In other words, the evaluators should be fully informed but independent.

Comparison of the influence on health will probably have to be made by anthropometric cross-sectional surveys in the two areas, as well as from infor-

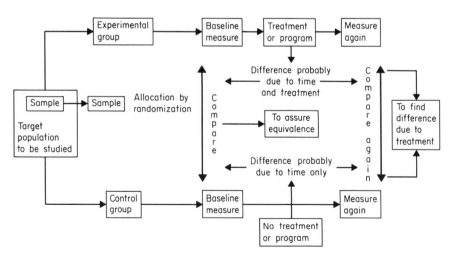

Figure 9-1 Ideal study design for making comparisons (modified from USAID, 1973).

mation from health services (''target hospitals'' or health centers), concerning the incidence of severe malnutrition and sometimes related deaths.

In areas in which the system is working, data can be obtained where growth monitoring has been initiated from service charts or other records retained at the clinic, in addition to the records kept by mothers (see Appendix A). In a trial situation, it may be best to review at intervals the percentage of young children of different ages ($<$ 1 year, 1 to 2 years, etc.) who are above or below various lines on the chart, or by using a plastic overlay with lines showing different levels (e.g., 80%, 70%, and 60% of reference weight for age) or by using a master card, kept in the clinic, on which children's weights are plotted (Fig. A-1) (Capone, 1970). In addition, the numbers of children with *unsatisfactory growth* of different types can be enumerated.

In addition, evaluation of other aspects (''operations research'') of the program have to be included, such as cost, logistics and coverage.

10
Training Program

The effect of the particular training program needs to be evaluated as regards trainees, trainers, and the attitudes and knowledge of the community, especially the mothers. Some aspects of such an evaluation process are given in Table 10-1.

Table 10-1 Evaluation at different levels

Community residents evaluate
Relevance of curriculum to perceived needs
Effect of training arrangements on trainees' relation to community and family
Effect of training on the health workers' ability to replace or supplement other health providers

Trainees evaluate
Convenience of training dates, duration, housing, etc.
Adequacy of per diem and other stipends
Relevance of curriculum to interests and perceived needs
Appropriateness of learning methods
Their own individual progress toward learning objectives

Trainers evaluate
Relevance of content to trainee needs
Relevance of methods to trainee learning capacities
Progress toward course objectives
Appropriateness of training materials
Progress of individual trainees
Adequacy of logistical arrangements
Reaction of trainees and community residents to training

Training supervisors and managers evaluate
Adherence of courses (methods, content and so forth) to plans and standards
Performance of individual trainers

Training designers evaluate
Appropriateness of content and methods to trainee needs and capacities
Appropriateness of training to field conditions and job requirements

Senior ministry of health personnel evaluate
The appropriateness of training strategies, including long-term skill development and training of associated personnel
The impact of training of community health workers effectiveness
Development of in-country training capacity
Effects of health workers on public health in their country

Donors evaluate everything listed, plus
Funding requests for individual courses
The work of external consultants

From World Federation of Public Health Associations, 1983b.

APPENDICES

Monitoring Community Child Nutrition

The word "monitoring" is not usually used to refer to groups of children, although it seems valid to do so. Essentially, the process consists of analyzing the numbers and percentages of children in different age groups being weighed falling into different levels during a defined period of time. Repeated collections of such information each year can give an approximate monitoring of the nutritional situation in the community served.

TECHNIQUES

Various methods can be used.

1. *Duplicate cards.* These can be filled in at the same time as the mother's card and retained at the clinic or by the weigher. They can be reviewed at intervals to assess the percentage of children below certain weight levels, with inadequate weight gains (by slope of growth lines), or both. This is usually not feasible.
2. *Master cards.* These were pioneered by Capone (1970) and successfully used in some parts of Africa (Capone, 1970), and a similar weight chart from Colombia could be used for the same purpose (Fig. A-1). Also, the WHO master card (Fig. A-2) can be employed in a similar way. All children attending during a specified period should have their weight plotted on the master card as well as on the usual card retained by the mother. Simple addition can give the number of children in various categories in different age groups, and percentages calculated.
3. *Tally sheet.* Alternatively, as in Kenya (CHANIS, 1986), a tally sheet may be used (Fig. A-3). This can be for selected age groups and each child's weight can be checked as normal weight (above line) or underweight (below line) for a period of 1 month. In the Kenya model, the "line" referred to is the lower line of a WHO-Morley type of graph (p. 21)—that is, the third centile for girls (approximately 80%). The age

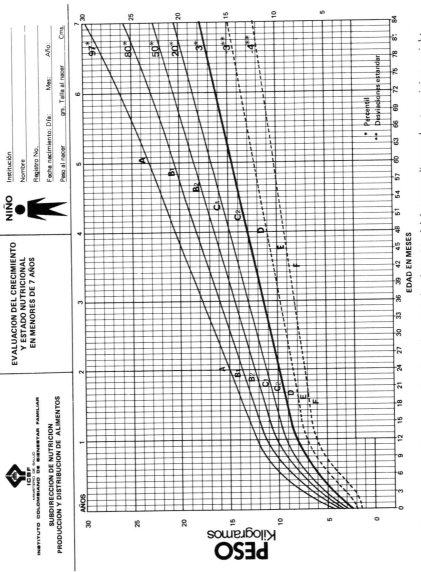

Figure A-1 Multizone weight chart (boys) (Colombia). Useful for recording and categorizing weight levels of children in a community (Institute of Family Welfare, Colombia). Retained in clinic and all weights plotted in specified period, enabling numbers and percentages in different zones to be calculated.

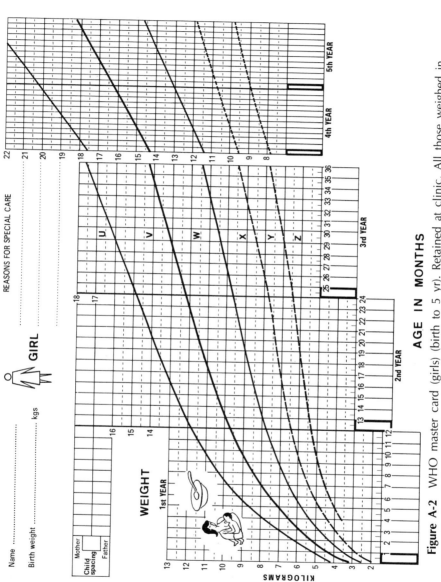

Figure A-2 WHO master card (girls) (birth to 5 yr). Retained at clinic. All those weighed in specified period are plotted and results calculated in each level.

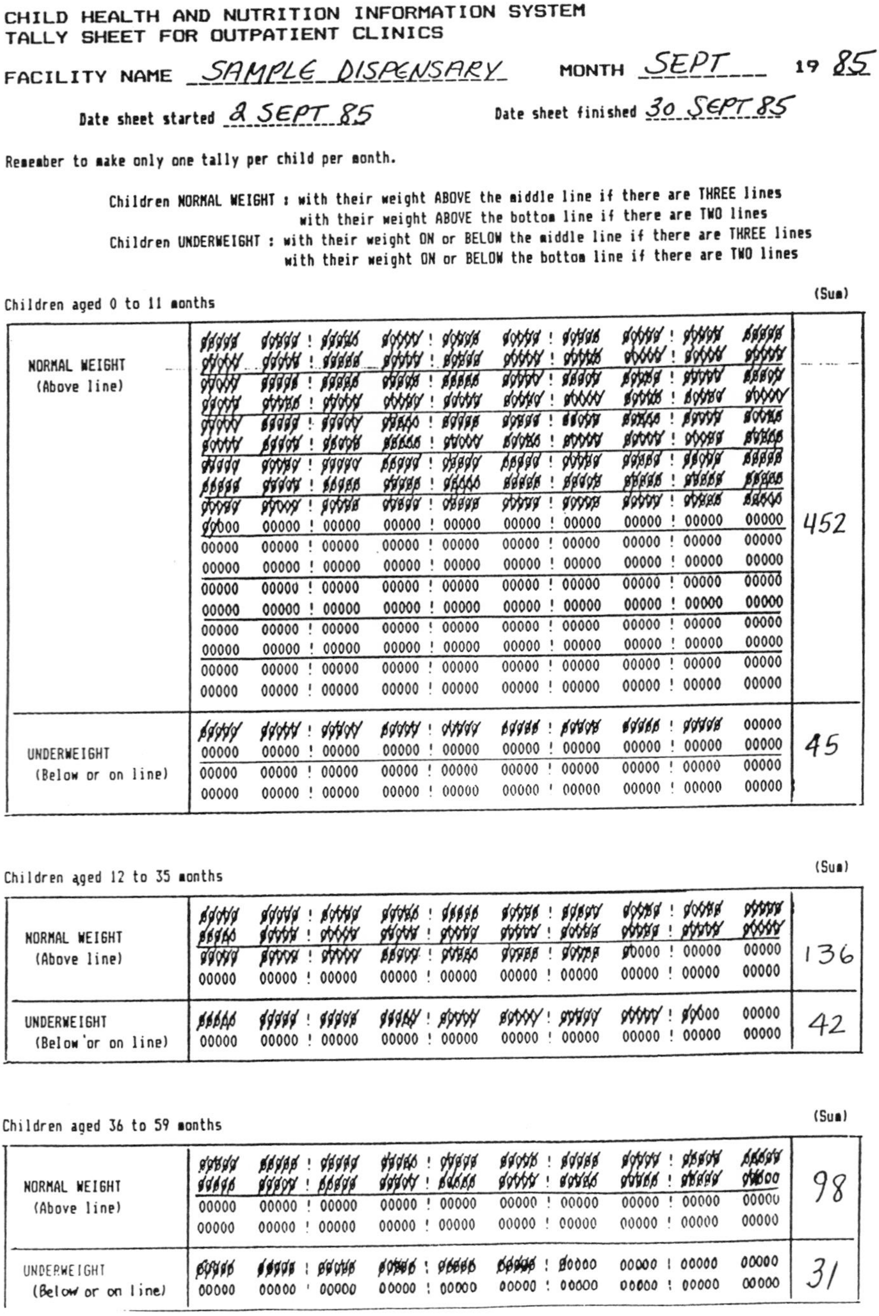

CHILD HEALTH AND NUTRITION INFORMATION SYSTEM
TALLY SHEET FOR OUTPATIENT CLINICS

FACILITY NAME __SAMPLE DISPENSARY__   MONTH _SEPT___ 19 85

Date sheet started _2 SEPT 85_   Date sheet finished _30 SEPT 85_

Remember to make only one tally per child per month.

Children NORMAL WEIGHT : with their weight ABOVE the middle line if there are THREE lines
                         with their weight ABOVE the bottom line if there are TWO lines
Children UNDERWEIGHT : with their weight ON or BELOW the middle line if there are THREE lines
                       with their weight ON or BELOW the bottom line if there are TWO lines

Children aged 0 to 11 months   (Sum)

| NORMAL WEIGHT (Above line) | | | | 452 |
| UNDERWEIGHT (Below or on line) | | | | 45 |

Children aged 12 to 35 months   (Sum)

| NORMAL WEIGHT (Above line) | | | | 136 |
| UNDERWEIGHT (Below or on line) | | | | 42 |

Children aged 36 to 59 months   (Sum)

| NORMAL WEIGHT (Above line) | | | | 98 |
| UNDERWEIGHT (Below or on line) | | | | 31 |

Figure A-3 Tally sheet used for recording weights of children in community studies (Kenya) (CHANIS, 1986).

100

groups selected in this model were 0 to 11 months, 12 to 35 months, and 36 to 59 months. Other age ranges might be more appropriate elsewhere.

REPORTING

For purposes of nontechnical reporting of results, it may be necessary to label all different categories used locally, such as "underweight," "*peso bajo,*" "second-degree malnutrition," and so forth.

A Point System for Comparative Evaluation of Weighing Scales*

These evaluation criteria, with several elaborations, are broadly laid out according to the general criteria established by a joint UNICEF and WHO meeting held June 24–26, 1985. The intention is to create criteria that will encompass diverse scale technologies (bar, tubular spring, circular spring, direct reading, and digital). Certain criteria are essential.

The weighted criteria for the various headings are:

1. Fundamental design	70 points	
2. Acceptability	50 points	
3. Scale error potential	40 points	
4. Operator error potential	50 points	
5. General criteria	60 points	
6. Sling/suspension	30 points	
Total value	300 points	

1. *Fundamental design:* 70 points

Maintenance: 15 points

Points of wear, fulcrum, rack and pinion, ability to prevent wear, other maintenance activities (see also fatigue).

Safety: 15 points

Scale hook strength, hanger hook strength, materials provided with scales, rope, hook (training for securing scale, scale stability, vertical, scale stability, pivoting, secured weights and counter weights, no sharp edge or roughness.

Durability: 15 points

Expected life, impact resistance, face material, body material, functional parts (electronic-only circuit integrity, source of power, alkaline, photo voltaic, lithium battery).

Portability: 10 points

Weight, compactness, handling ease.

Universality: 10 points

*From Burns and Rohde, 1988.

Babies 0 to 6 months, infants 6 to 24 months, toddlers 24 to 36 months, children 36 to 60 months, mothers.

Tare: 5 points

Number of kilograms of tare (scope of tare).

2. *Acceptability:* 50 points

   Operator: 20 points

   Ease of reading, ease of operating, weighing time, ease of transporting, perceived safety, time to tare, tools to tare.

   Mother: 20 points

   Nonthreatening appearance, cultural acceptability of suspending a child, perceived safety, apprehension, comprehension of weighing mechanism.

   Child: 10 points

   Apprehension, discomfort.

3. *Scale error potential:* 40 points

   Accuracy: (sine qua non plus or minus 100 grams or less).

   Temperature compensation, hysteresis, creep (a form of stretch with loading).

   Linearity:

   The ability to measure with the same accuracy over a range of weights.

   Precision:

   Consistency of reading.

   Sensitivity:

   Least weight to cause movement.

   Unobvious damage:

   Damage to rack and pinion, damage to springs, damage to weight.

   Fatigue:

   Spring wear, other fatigue, fulcrum wear.

4. *Operator error potential:* 50 points

   Accuracy: 15 points

   Clarity of markings/read out; simplicity; no complicated calculations; errors of transposition (scale to chart); ability to specify language.

   Tare:

   Accuracy of taring, loss of tare during weighing.

   Parallax: 5 points

   Closeness of indicator to slide, closeness of needle to face.

   Complexity of use: 15 points

   Number of hands needed to weigh, number of movements to weigh (see acceptability).

   Damping: 10 points

   Accurately read with child in motion.

   Self-contained: 5 points

   Number of detached parts of loose hooks and weights.

5. *General criteria:* 40 points

   Cost: 30 points

   Real cost, cost of packing, shadow costing value of in-country production, additional costs for special training.

Packaging: 5 points
Unit packing, pack to specifications.

Potential for local manufacture: 5 points

Instructions: 10 points
Use, assembly, local language, illustration.

6. *Sling/Suspension:* 30 points
(Stand-on scale receives 30 points automatically.)

Operator: 10 points
Ease of suspension, ease of putting child in sling, slinging time, ease of transporting, perceived safety, cleanliness.

Mother: 10 points
Nonthreatening appearance, cultural acceptability, perceived safety, apprehension.

Child: 10 points
Comfort of sling, nonconfining sling, size of leg holds (child), head rest (infant), grasp of dimensions, feel of material.

APPENDIX C

Focus Group Interviews*

Focus group interviews or exploratory group sessions are a qualitative research technique frequently utilized in social science research. A focus group meeting is a discussion in which a small group of informants (6 to 12 people), guided by a facilitator or moderator, talk freely and spontaneously about themes considered important to the investigation. The participants are chosen from a target group whose opinions and ideas are of interest to the research. Usually more than one group session is needed to assure good coverage. Sessions can be conducted with various subgroups within the target population. Participants may be recruited at random and briefly interviewed to determine if they qualify for the group.

Focus groups could be utilized in a study of health-seeking behavior to:

1. Focus the research and formulate questions for the formal interview questionnaire.
2. Supplement the information on community knowledge, beliefs, attitudes, and perceptions about health and health resources.
3. Develop research hypotheses for additional studies.
4. Develop vocabularies for health education programs.

A typical focus group for this research would be comprised of health providers, health center personnel, rural health promoters, midwives, pharmacists, and so forth. Another might be mothers of children under 5 years of age.

The focus group meeting is usually tape-recorded, although an observer (recorder) also takes notes on the discussion. An open conversation takes place in which each participant has the opportunity to speak, ask questions of other participants, and respond to the comments of others, including the facilitator. Interaction among the participants is stimulated by the discussion of various themes relevant to the research. The facilitator guides the sessions so that all subjects of interest are covered.

A focus group session typically lasts up to 1½ hours. Generally, the first

*Excerpted with permission from Scrimshaw and Hurtado, 1987. Videotape of procedures available from Dr. S. Scrimshaw, School of Public Health, University of California, Los Angeles, CA 90024.

sessions are longer than the following ones because all of the information is new. Thereafter, the facilitator is able to move the discussion along more quickly over the points that have been treated by the other groups, when it is clear that all the groups have the same opinion. The number of focus group sessions to be conducted depends on project needs, resources, and whether new information is still forthcoming (i.e., whether contrasting views from various groups in the community are still emerging).

The location for the focus group meeting should be one where the participants feel comfortable talking openly and should be neutral in terms of the interests of the investigation. For example, the community health center is not an appropriate place for meetings about local medical beliefs or the use of different health resources. The parish or municipal hall would be a more appropriate choice.

PREPARATION FOR THE FOCUS GROUP SESSION

For the focus group session to be most productive, participants should be of the same sex, age group, and socioeconomic background (ethnic group, marital status, educational level, etc.). Invitations to participate are extended about 1 week or several days in advance. Atlhough not always feasible, recruiting participants using a random sample is the preferred method. The following steps can be followed when inviting the participants.

1. Talk about something of interest to the potential participant (the children, the climate, the marketplace, etc.)
2. In a sincere way tell the participant about the institution sponsoring the study and the general purpose of the visit to the community.
3. Explain the nature of the meeting planned and invite the person to participate along with neighbors and others in the community. Do not indicate the specific subject of the session in advance. Mention names of some of those who have volunteered to come. (This is not done for some focus groups where respondents do not know each other.)
4. Confirm the date, time, and place of the meeting, how long it will last, and that refreshments will be served.
5. If the person does not wish to participate, or cannot, emphasize the importance of contributions by all. If the person still declines, express your thanks and leave.
6. If the individual is interested in participating, confirm the day, hour, and place, and make a brief statement about the importance of participation and of being punctual so that others are not kept waiting.

The Facilitator

The facilitator uses a discussion guide or outline to keep the session focused. The guide incorporates the objectives of the study, and usually includes general open-ended questions (e.g., ''What do people here do?'' instead of ''What do you do?''). (See sample guide in original.)

The points listed next outline the role of the facilitator.

1. Introduce the discussion topics. The facilitator does not need to be an expert on each topic being discussed, but should be familiar enough with the subject matter to pose relevant questions. The facilitator should not convey the impression of being an expert. From the outset, adopt an enthusiastic, lively approach to help put the participants at ease. Maintain a sense of humor.

2. Lead the group; do not be led by it. Formulate appropriate questions and react suitably and neutrally to the comments. Emphasize that there is no right or wrong answer. Gestures and other nonverbal forms of communication (a nod or shake of the head) should not suggest agreement or disagreement with the participants' comments. Avoid reacting to the discussion or expressing personal opinions that could influence the participants. Be aware of personal biases and prejudices and refrain from asking more questions of a person whose ideas are in accord with yours.

3. Observe the participants and be conscious of the extent of their involvement and their reactions. Encourage all to participate and do not allow a few individuals to monopolize the discussion. (Refer to the group management techniques discussed later in original.)

4. Listen carefully in order to move the discussion logically from point to point and to relate participants' comments to the next question (e.g., ''your point about how long you have to wait at clinics reminds me that I wanted to ask you where you go if you don't have time to go to the clinic''). Guide the meeting away from a question/answer, interviewer/interviewee session toward a more egalitarian group discussion so that the participants communicate among themselves, forgetting the presence of the facilitator.

5. Build rapport with the participants and gain their confidence and trust in order to probe their responses and comments more deeply.

6. Empathize with the participants and be able to understand not only what they say but also what it means to them. Take a sincere interest in the participants and in learning about them.

7. Be flexible and open to suggestions, changes, interruptions, and lack of participation.

8. Subtly control the time allotted to each question and to the meeting in general, without seeming to be watching the clock or rushing the participants.

9. Control the rhythm of the meeting. For example, the conversation should move quickly over issues that have been discussed by other groups, if the facilitator is sure that the group has expressed the same opinion as the others. New information or opinions, however, should be discussed in depth. For this reason the first focus group session to take place is usually the longest.

10. Observe the participants' nonverbal communication and respond accordingly. For example, the way an individual is seated, gestures, and other movements supplement verbal communication and may suggest impatience, tranquility, fatigue, boredom, anxiety, and the like.
11. Be aware of your tone of voice. An overly assertive, aggressive, or imperative tone can intimidate the participants, particularly in the case of probing questions, those that are asked several times. It might seem that the participant is being attacked if the tone of voice sounds unfriendly.

The recorder is present, primarily as an observer, during the focus group session and is responsible for taking notes on the discussion. The notes should include the following points.

1. Date of the meeting and the time it began and ended.
2. The name of the community and a brief description of it, and any other information that may bear on the activities of the participants (e.g., the distance from the community to the next largest town or political unit).
3. The place where the meeting is being held, a brief description of it, and information on how the location could affect the participants (is it large enough, comfortable, conveniently located, etc.).
4. The number of participants and some descriptive data on them, such as sex, approximate age, and other kinds of information important to the study (e.g., number of women whose children have/have not been vaccinated, who use/do not use family planning methods).
5. A general description of the group dynamics, the level of participation, whether there is a dominant participant, interest level (fatigue, anxiety, boredom, etc.).
6. The interruptions and distractions that occur during the meeting.
7. What makes the participants laugh, what seems to make them reluctant to answer, how the discussion is ended.
8. The opinions of the participants, using phrases such as: The majority of the group is of the opinion that . . . but Mrs. Smith . . . said the group is divided in the middle; some think that. . . . The recorder should use quotation marks to indicate the participants' own words. Personal impressions and observations should be noted in parentheses. The tape recording of the meeting will help the recorder amplify notes taken during the sessions. (The recorder is responsible for operating the tape recorder.)
9. The general vocabulary of the participants. The recorder should make an effort to note the participants' own words, in the local language. (Remember that one goal of the research is to learn as many local expressions as possible.)

Although it is the facilitator's responsibility to direct the discussion and moderate the meeting, the recorder may participate, with discretion, especially in the following situations.

1. Occasionally, the facilitator may miss comments made by one person while listening to another. In that case the recorder can say, for example, "Mrs. Smith mentioned something that we did not hear. Could you repeat what you said, Mrs. Smith?"
2. The recorder can suggest a new question or topic important to the study.
3. In the event the facilitator has omitted a question from the guide, the recorder can point this out. (Both the recorder and the facilitator should have a copy of the discussion guide at the meetings.)
4. The recorder should note that the facilitator has lost control of the meeting.
5. The recorder can suggest ways to make the discussion more meaningful.
6. The recorder can help the facilitator resolve internal conflicts.

THE FOCUS GROUP SESSION

Before the Meeting

The facilitator and the recorder should be the first to arrive, on time, at the meeting place. They should start talking informally with the participants as they arrive or with other curious individuals who may have gathered. Take advantage of this time to learn people's names and something of their interests. Generally, almost all will avoid being "the first to arrive" and will wait until they see others arriving. Therefore, it is important to give the impression that all is ready to begin.

The facilitator should assure that the seating arrangement will encourage all participants to talk. It is recommended that the participants sit in a circle, more or less at the same distance from the facilitator. The facilitator should make sure that there are no interruptions from outside the group once the session begins. Ideally, the facilitator and the participants should be of the same sex.

Materials needed for a group session include a tape recorder, blank cassettes, batteries (where no electricity is available), and discussion guides.

Opening the Meeting

The introduction to a focus group meeting is a key moment because it determines tone and atmosphere. As the meeting begins, the facilitator should be animated and chatty to put the participants at ease. In the introduction, the facilitator should include the following points.

1. Make the introductions and explain the roles of the facilitator and recorder.
2. Ask the participants to give their names (last names not necessary). The facilitator should learn the names quickly and use them when speaking to the participants.

3. Explain that the meeting is not intended to be an educational lecture, but an effort to gather opinions and ideas from the group for the purpose of incorporating them into a health program, educational campaign, and so on. The facilitator also explains that the meeting has been arranged to learn from the participants, that the facilitator and recorder are not experts on the subject.
4. Point out that the opinions of all participants are important and that all should feel free to express themselves on the subjects discussed.
5. Explain that the only rules of the meeting are that the speaker should address the subject being discussed and that only one person should speak at a time.
6. Start the meeting by asking each participant a general question not related to the topic to be discussed. That way everyone will have an opportunity to speak about a neutral subject at the beginning of the meeting (e.g., the facilitator can ask how many children each participants has or how many years each has lived in the village)

Focus Group Management Techniques

Several easy-to-learn techniques can be applied to the management of a focus group. These are particularly helpful in determining the subjects to be discussed and the specific questions to be asked.

Clarification

After a participant answers a question the facilitator can repeat the response in the form of a question for clarification or to encourage further discussion (e.g., "Can you tell me more about . . . ?" or "What do you mean when you say . . . ?").

Substitution

A question can be rephrased using different words, but without altering the original meaning. The facilitator should be sure that the way the question is formulated does not hint at the answer (e.g., "Until what age are children suckled here?" or "How long do you breast-feed your infants here?").

Reorientation

To keep the discussion lively and interesting, a reorientation technique can be effective. The facilitator can use one participant's response or comment to re-state the question for someone else [e.g., "Mrs. Smith, you tell us that you breast-feed until the age of 6 months. And you, Mrs. Jones (who has not given an opinion), until what age do you breast-feed your children?"].

The Expert

It is recommended that the "specialist" or "expert," like the health promoter, the midwife, or someone with authority, such as the mayor, not be present at focus group meetings unless the meeting is scheduled specifically to include their participation. Nevertheless, if their attendance is unavoidable, explain to them, before the meeting, that the best way for them to contribute is to *listen* to the discussion and then share their ideas and conclusions with the facilitator *after* the meeting.

The Dominant Participant

When the group has a dominant participants, the facilitator must try to elicit more contributions from the others in attendance. It is also possible to change the subject and to avoid eye contact with the dominant participant in order to discourage that individual from speaking. If all else fails, the facilitator can politely request that the others be allowed to speak.

The Reluctant Participant

To encourage a quiet participant to contribute more to the discussion, the facilitator should direct attention to that person using the individual's name and openly asking for an opinion. The participant can make more eye contact with the reluctant participant, thus encouraging greater contribution. It is possible to ask the participant to comment on what another person has said or to summarize what the group has said about a particular subject.

Additional Techniques

An effective way to achieve maximum group participation is for the facilitator to write down the kinds of information needed on the subject and explain the need for knowledge to the group. The participants will feel good about being able to assist and will recognize the value of their personal experiences.

Also, one can use photographs or pictures to stimulate discussion. For example, show a picture of a malnourished child and ask, "How does this child look (ill, healthy)? What should the child's mother do? If she were your neighbor, what would you advise her to do?"

Results from a previous study can be presented for discussion.

Ending the Meeting

To conclude the focus group meeting, the facilitator should:

1. Explain that the meeting is about to end, ask the participants to think about what has been discussed, and ask them one by one if they have any other comments. The relevant comments can be explored in greater depth.
2. Thank the participants for their contributions and reaffirm that their ideas have been valuable and will be used in the program planning, design, educational materials, and the like, as appropriate to the project.
3. Listen for additional comments while refreshments are served (if any).

After the group session the facilitator and recorder must meet to review and complete the notes taken during the meeting.

Introducing the Concept
of Weighing in a Village*

Introduced in workshops in Indonesia. Different techniques may be needed in other cultures.

Setting: A community center, school, home, or shaded area outside.

Time: Half a day.

Purpose: To assist villagers in recognizing the extent of nutrition problems in their community and to encourage mothers to weigh their children as a way of knowing whether the children are healthy.

Preparation: Meet with village leaders to explain the purpose of the activity.

Invite the villagers or representatives of the village to attend, being sure to include mothers and 15 to 20 children under 5 years of age.

You will need a weighing scale and a large poster of a weight chart. If these are not easily available locally, check with UNICEF or the ministry of health.

Procedure:

1. Allow the village leader to introduce the group.
2. Explain the purpose of the visit.
3. Show the villagers the picture of the healthy child. Ask, "Is this child healthy? How many children in our community are healthy? Are there many children who are not very healthy? How can we know which children are not very healthy?"
4. Ask the villagers if they would like to survey the children to know if they are healthy. In this way we can make a picture or graph of the health situation of children in our village. If the villagers are interested, proceed by explaining that weight is one indication of health. Talk about how a child's weight should increase with age.
5. Ask for a volunteer. Weigh the child and mark the weight on the chart. Proceed with the other children. Mark each weight on the graph.
6. When the children all have been weighed, explain the graph to the villagers. How is the health situation for these children? What about the other children? Would they like to weigh all of the children in the community? Explain that by identifying how many children are in danger of

*From Srinivasan, 1982.

poor health, the community can plan to take action to solve the problem.
7. Close the meeting on a positive note. Encourage parents by telling them that they can help their children to be healthy. Give a few simple practical suggestions.

This is a good way to involve villagers in their own village analysis. Leave the chart in the community center and repeat the activity after 6 months to help the village evaluate community progress in eliminating malnutrition.

In order to make the meeting proceed more quickly you may want to weigh a sample of the children in the village before the meeting. Plot the weights on the graph during the meeting.

Basic Dietary Messages:
Improving Young Child Growth*

Key points to remember are:

- Well babies less than 4 months old need no other milk or food apart from breastmilk.
- Adding oil, margarine, or sugar and milk, eggs or groundnuts makes *uji* (local porridge) energy rich and helps young children grow well.
- Feed often—small children have small stomachs.
- Feed older children at least three times a day and given them snacks between meals.
- Breast-feed until child is 2 years old.
- Feed sick children something and give extra food when they recover.

*From Child Health and Information System (CHANIS), Health Information Unit, Ministry of Health, Nairobi, Kenya, 1986.

Nutrition Education Messages*

Clear, specific, geared to common foods, culturally acceptable.

A. Children of 0 to 3 months whose weight does not increase during one month.

Advice:
1. The child should be breastfed three to five times more often than usual every day.
   Note: The more frequently a baby is breastfed the more the mother's milk production will increase. Do not worry, mother's milk will not be "exhausted" if it is given often.
2. A breast-feeding mother should drink an extra two glasses of fresh water three times daily.
   Note: To increase the volume of mother's milk, the mother should drink more. Cooking water from small green peas or other beans or soup made from vegetables are also good for additional drinks.
3. In case there is a well-known herb (traditional medicine) known to increase the flow of mother's milk, it should be suggested to be used.
   Note: In order to improve the flow of mother's milk, the mother herself should believe that she is able to breast-feed her baby. The use of Jamu (herbal tea) or other habits that have become a tradition in the area concerned will make a mother more confident that she is able to nurse her baby well. This belief has a positive influence on the production of mother's milk (ASI).

B. Children of 0 to 3 months of age whose weight does not increase two months in succession.

Repeat advice given the previous month. Make inquiries as to whether or not all advice given was carried out and, if not, ask what the problems were. Then give the additional advice: The mother should eat two dishes of food more than she usually eats in a day.

*From UPGK, The Indonesia Experience, Sukmanah, 1987.

Note: A nursing mother should eat for two persons: for herself and the baby she is nursing. For this reason, she has to eat more than usual. Food should consist of a staple food and side dishes. The other members of the family can be asked to help remind the mother that she should eat more and, if necessary, put aside part of their food for mothers.

C. Children of 3 to 7 months whose weight does not increase during one month.

Advice:
Give the child one medium-size dish of porridge three times a day.
Note: Mother's milk is still important, but the child also needs additional food. Porridge can be made of rice. Add mashed *tempeh* or *tahu* to the porridge. If the child seems to have already been given porridge three times every day, give one more dish a day.

D. Children of 3 to 7 months whose weight does not increase two months in succession.

Repeat advice given last month. Make inquiries as to whether or not all advice given was carried out and, if not, ask what the problems were. Then the following advice is given: give the child porridge five times a day, each time one given a medium-size dish as the portion.

E. Children of 7 to 12 months whose weight does not increase during one month.

Advice:
Apart from porridge given five times a day (each time one medium-size dish of porridge), also give the child rice twice a day with mashed side dishes.
Note: Do not hesitate to give your child such food frequently. A child of this age needs a lot of food. However, due to its small stomach, food should be given frequently. In the meantime nursing should be continued. It is advisable that mother's milk be given after food and not before. This is intended not to make the child feel satisfied during the meal.

F. Children of 7 to 12 months whose weight does not increase two months in succession.

Repeat advice given last month. Make inquiries as to whether or not all advice given was carried out and, if not, what the problems were. Then give new advice: apart from five to six dishes of food every day, a child should be given snacks.

Note: At this age a child tends to put anything into its mouth. Give the infant a snack, something for it to hold, which at the same time constitutes very useful additional food. Fried *tempeh* (fungus-digested soya product) or sweet potato prepared by the mother at home are cheap and healthy foods. Be sure not to make it a habit to give your infant unhealthy snacks such as ice, candies, and the like.

G. Children of 12 to 24 months whose weight does not increase during one month.

Advice:
Give the child adult food five times a day.
Note: This child is already big and needs food used by adults. The child, however, should eat more frequently than adults do. Be sure that such food consists of rice, side dishes, *tahu tempeh,* tari fish, and vegetables. Side dishes cooked with *santan* (coconut milk) and fried side dishes are very good for children. Make sure that there is variety in the dishes served so that the child does not get bored. Nursing should be continued until the child is 2 years old.

H. Children of 12 to 24 months whose weight does not increase two months in succession.

Repeat advice given last month. Make inquiries as to whether or not all advice given was carried out and if not what the problems were. Then give new advice: restore the appetite of the child by changing the kind of food offered.

Note: Suggest also that the mother gives food that the child likes. Sometimes, by having a meal together with other children, the child will want to eat.

I. Children of 24 months and older whose weight does not increase during one month.

Advice:
The child should eat half as much as his or her father eats.
Note: In order to be sure that the child gets this volume of food, put aside the child's portion in a separate dish. It is advisable that the father encourage his child to consume the entire portion put aside for him or her.

J. Children of 24 months and older whose weight does not increase two months in succession.

Repeat advice given last month. Make inquiries as to whether or not all advice given was carried out and if not what the problems were. Then give new advice: once a day a child should eat together with other children.
Note: By having a joint meal with other children, the child is encouraged to eat more. If this is done every day, the child will get used to eating more.

Comparative Systems: Descriptive Accounts*

There are many different approaches to growth monitoring and promotion (GMP) activities that are carried out within health delivery. Here are several approaches that are considered promising in terms of their high coverage, comprehensive promotion of action, and positive effect on nutrition and health status. The entry points for growth monitoring vary in each of these examples.

DOMINICAN REPUBLIC—A HOME/COMMUNITY-BASED PROGRAM

A monthly home visit is the key entry point of the CARITAS Dominicana/ Catholic Relief Service Applied Nutrition Education Program in the Dominican Republic. Monthly activities of the program, which began in September 1983, reached more than 85% of the population with children under 5 years in 70 communities throughout the country by 1986. Significant changes in the knowledge of appropriate feeding practices resulted. When the program began, the level of stage 2 and 3 malnutrition (moderate to severe malnutrition) was over 14%. Three years later that figure was more than halved to below 7% among children in the program.

Program success increased with the following: the selection of communities at high risk to malnutrition; careful selection and permanent, ongoing training of personnel; continuous supervision for technical and motivational purposes; a well-defined and implemented GMP/nutrition education intervention; effective communication strategies that emphasized program prestige in the communities; and a simple and effective information system for internal surveillance and ongoing evaluation.

ECUADOR—HEALTH CENTER-BASED PROGRAM

Ecuador's PEM-PAAMI nutrition program, funded by AID in two provinces, used weighing to screen for food supplements. It is currently being broadened

*From Teller, Yee, & Zerfas, 1987.

118

and integrated with other child survival actions, including a pilot project to bring mothers into the rural health centers for growth monitoring and group and individualized nutrition counseling. An integrated set of child survival services is available at the centers, as well as curative treatment by social service doctors. Mothers have learned to understand the improved growth chart and to improve certain health and nutrition behaviors.

A locally produced substitute for imported supplementary or weaning food has been developed and favorably tested. The program, which began in 1984, has been expanded nationally and incorporated into the campaigns of the national child survival program. Over 60% of the children under age 2 were weighed in the growth monitoring campaign in mid-1986.

Nutrition education and training materials have been developed and mass media campaigns are being carried out. The program is still being improved, and the reports are promising.

THAILAND: COMMUNITY-BASED PRIMARY HEALTH CARE

The quarterly nutritional surveillance rally held at a common meeting point in the village is the entry point for primary health care in most of Thailand. Growth monitoring is usually done by village health volunteers under the supervision of Ministry of Health officers. Nutrition education and targeted supplementary feeding with locally produced weaning foods are provided. Approximately 50% of the children under 5 years in 37,000 villages in Thailand are now in the nutrition surveillance program. The data generated are used for targeting monthly home visits of malnourished children and community and district health and development planning purposes. Moderate and severe malnutrition was reduced by 50% between 1982 and 1985, and the nutrition program is believed to have played a major role.

UNICEF feels that the Thai program may be the first successful example of growth monitoring being done properly and making a difference on a national scale. This is the result of political commitment at the top, as well as social mobilization at the provincial and district levels and ongoing community development.

INDONESIA—VILLAGE MOTHERS MEETINGS

In 1981, 7000 trained field-workers and a network of village family planning posts staffed by thousands of volunteers were used to help expand the government's family nutrition improvement program in 15,000 villages on the islands of Java and Bali.

The centerpiece of the campaign is a rainbow-colored growth chart specially designed after intensive research. The main message of the process was that monthly weight gain in children is good, a constant weight is a warning sign, and weight loss is a danger sign.

The traditional village mothers meeting place was used as the weighing point. Children under 3 years were weighed each month with a common marketplace scale and the results entered by the mother. On the reverse side of the chart, panels contained information on how to make oral rehydration salts and nutritious weaning foods.

The growth chart was kept in the home by the mother, thus instilling in the mother the responsibility for good nutrition. Because the chart made the child's growth visible and readable for the mother, it was a powerful educational and communication channel for informing mothers of the relationship among food, illness, weight gain, and health.

According to UNICEF's 1986–1987 *State of the World's Children* publications, 5 million Indonesian mothers now regularly weigh their children and check on their growth, with children under 5 years regularly attending the monthly weighing sessions. Up to 2.5 million children are being weighed regularly at 124,000 growth monitoring centers established in two-thirds of the nation's villages. Evaluation reports show children weighing in at a consistently higher weight. Several case studies show that weighing has become a popular community activity and that nutrition awareness has soared. The message that "weight gain is good" is well understood and accepted, and communities have organized group activities to promote good nutrition as part of the growth monitoring session.

TAMIL NADU, INDIA—MIXED HOME AND FACILITY BASED

This large-scale growth monitoring and targeted supplemental feeding program focuses on children 6 to 36 months of age in 9000 villages. Children in the program who are diagnosed as malnourished are given supplemental feedings. In a recent book by the World Bank entitled *Malnutrition: What Can Be Done?*, author Alan Berg notes that 2 years after the program was established, the number of children in the program who were not growing adequately and required feeding fell by 57%—even during a year of a bad drought. By December 1986, there was a 53% decline in serious and severe malnutrition among children in the project.

Growth of over 90% of the children in the program is monitored monthly. Total cost per child for weighing and supplementary feeding along with the related nutrition education is less than $12 per year. One very encouraging sign is among children who were once in the program. By the age of 5, those children are almost 4 pounds heavier than those from control villages.

Acknowledgments

WORKSHOP PARTICIPANTS

Grateful thanks are due to the International Workshop held at the Caribbean Food and Nutrition Institute, Jamaica (May 1987). Participants in attendance and corresponding are as indicated.

IUNS Working Group II/1: Growth Monitoring and Nutrition Action

Chairperson: Derrick Jelliffe (USA)
Deputy Chairperson: Luis Fajardo (Colombia)
Members: Michael Gurney (WHO), Lukas Hendrata (UNICEF), Ron Israel (USA),*
G. Ibn Auf Suliamn (Sudan),* W. Klaver (Netherlands),* T.N. Maletnlema (Tanzania),* David Morley (U.K.), Alberto Pradilla (WHO), Dinesh Sinha (CFNI, Jamaica), Alfred Zerfas (Australia)

IUNS Committee IV/6: Nutrition Education and Training of Nurses and Auxiliary Health Workers

Chairperson: Patrice Jelliffe (USA)
Deputy Chairperson: Mary Ann Small Capistrano (Brazil)*
Members: Luzmilla de Illueca (Panama),* Samiarti Martosewojo (Indonesia),* Amelia Salomon (Chile),* Eunice K. Kithinji (Kenya),* Helen F. McGrane (USA),* Manuelita Zephirin (CFNI, Barbados)*

International Agencies

CFNI (Caribbean Food and Nutrition Institute, Jamaica): A. Wynante Patterson
PAHO (Pan American Health Organization): Carlos Daza
Ministry of Health, Indonesia: Titi Sukmanah

CORRESPONDENTS

In addition, sincere thanks are due to the following for offering valuable advice at different times: Mr. D. J. Alnwick, Regional Nutrition Adviser, UNICEF East African

*Corresponding participants.

Regional Office, Nairobi, Kenya; Dr. C. Goplan, Director, Nutrition Foundation of India, New Delhi, India; Dr. Shanti Ghosh, New Delhi, India; Ms. Marcia Griffiths, Manoff International, Inc., New York, USA; Dr. R. Goodwin, The Health Centre, Kirkwall, Orkney, New Scotland, U.K.; Ms. Susan Hewes de Calderon, Roosevelt Hospital, Guatemala City, Guatemala; Dr. Wijnand Klaver, International Cause in Food Service and Nutrition, Wageningen, The Netherlands; Professor Y. Hofvander, International Child Health, Medical School, University of Uppsala, Sweden; Dr. Nicholas Luykx, Deputy Division, Office of Nutrition, USAID, Washington, D.C., USA; Dr. D. Nabarro, London School of Hygiene and Tropical Medicine, London, U.K.; Dr. M. Pechevis, International Children's Centre, Paris, France; Dr. Charles Teller, International Nutrition Unit, Logical Technical Services, Inc., Washington, D.C., USA.

COVER DESIGN AND ILLUSTRATIONS

The symbolic design on the cover indicating the need for community involvement is reproduced courtesy of A. Fugelsang from his book, *Applied Communications in Developing Countries* (1973). Grateful thanks are due to Suzanne Westman for assistance with the illustrations.

Bibliography*

Aarons, A., and Hawes, H. (1979). *Child-to-child.* Macmillan, London.

Abel, R. (1986) *Trop. Doctor, 6,* 45. Traditional beliefs against weighing children regularly.

*Abbatt, F. R. (1980). *Teaching for better learning.* A guide for primary health care staff. WHO, Geneva.

Agency for International Development (1972). *Evaluation handbook.* Suppl. 11. USAID, Washington, D.C.

Alam, N., Wojtyniak, B., and Mujibun Rahman, M. (1989). *Amer. J. Clin. Nutr., 49,* 884. Anthropometric indicators and risk of death.

Anderson, M. (1979). *Amer. J. Clin. Nutr. 32,* 2339. Comparison of anthropometric measures of nutrition status in pre-school children in five developing countries.

American Home Economics Association (1977). *Working with villagers: Trainers manual and prototype lessons.* Washington, D.C.

Arole, M. (1988). *Indian J. Ped., 55,* 100. A comprehensive approach to community welfare: Growth monitoring and the role of women in Jamkhed.

Baker, J. (1986). Operations research: A tool for strengthening and expansion of child growth. Working Paper No. 8. UNICEF, New Delhi.

Barbero, G. J., and McKay, R. J. (1979). Failure to thrive. In *Nelson's Textbook of Pediatrics,* 11th edition, edited by V. C. Vaughan, R. J. McKay, and R. E. Behrman, pp. 311–312. W. B. Samuels, Philadelphia.

Barclay, E. J., and Van Der Vynckt, S. (1984). Easy-to-make teaching aids. Nutrition Education Series No. 10. UNESCO, Paris.

Berg, A. (1987). *Malnutrition: What can be done?* Johns Hopkins University Press, Baltimore.

Berggren, G., Michele, D., Guyer, M., and Whitaker, M. (1986). Training and training modules in monitoring and promotion of child growth with focus on primary level workers. UNICEF Meeting, New Delhi.

Briend, A., Wojtyniak, B., and Rowland, M. G. M. (1987). *Lancet, ii,* 725. Arm circumference and other factors in children at high risk of death in rural Bangladesh.

*Not all references are quoted in the text. Additional lists of references can be obtained from The Clearinghouse on Infant and Maternal Nutrition, APHA, International Health Programs, 1015 Fifteenth St. N.W., Washington, D.C. 20005. Suggested publications for a growth monitoring library are indicated by an asterisk (*). These are intended for use when considering the introduction or modification of growth monitoring systems.

Brunetto, A. L., and Pearson, A. D. J. (1988). *J. Trop. Ped., 34,* 22. Health education: Parents' perceptions.

Burns, J. D., Carrière, R. C., and Rohde, J. E. (1988). *Ind. J. Ped., 55,* Suppl. 1, S.26. Growth chart design.

Burns, J. D., and Rohde, J. E. (1988). *Ind. J. Ped., 55,* Suppl. 1, S.31. Weighing scales: Design and choices.

Campbell, J. L., Cutting, W. A. M., Elton, R. A., Minton, E. J., and Spreng, J. (1985) *Trans. Roy. Soc. Trop. Med. Hyg., 79,* 409. The portable Nabarro weight-height anthropometric nutrition assessment chart: A field trial in three countries in Africa.

Capone, C. (1970). Master chart for centre analysis of weight levels. Catholic Relief Services, Nairobi.

Carrington, M. E., Griffiths, M., and Diamond, M. (1987). Guide to mass media and support materials for nutrition education in developing countries. INCS/EDC, Newton, Mass.

CHANIS (Child Health Information and Nutrition Information System) (1986). Health Information Unit, Ministry of Health, Nairobi.

Chaudhuri, S. N. (1988). *Ind. J. Ped., 55,* Suppl. 1, S.84. Growth monitoring in the evolution of clinic based health care through a community based action programme.

CONTACT (December 7, 1987). Health teaching stories.

Cowan, B. (1988). *Ind. J. Ped., 55,* Suppl. 1. Growth monitoring as a critical means to provide primary health care.

Da Cunha, G. (1986). Child growth and social marketing. Notes for a preparatory consultation. *Working Document* No. 4 (1186F/11). UNICEF, New York.

Davies, D. P., and Leung, S. (1984). *Hong Kong J. Pediat., 1,* 3. Patterns of early weight gain in Chinese babies.

Dowling, M. A. C., and Ritson, R. (1987). Human resources for health. WHO/Educ. 88.193.

Essex, B., and Gosling, H. (1987). Nutrition and the community health worker. Guidelines for decision-making. Paper presented at WHO/IUNS Workshop, Caribbean Food and Nutrition Institute, Jamaica, March 10–18, 1987.

Feuerstein, M. T. (1986). *Partners in evaluation.* Evaluating development and community programmes with participants. Macmillan, London.

Food and Agriculture Organization (1981). Guidelines for curriculum content for agricultural training in South-East Asia. Food Policy and Nutrition Division, FAO, Rome.

Forsyth, S. J. (1984). *Food & Nutrition Bull., 6,* 22. Nutrition education: Lack of success in teaching Papua New Guinea mothers to distinguish "good" from "not good" weight development charts.

Foundation for Indonesian Welfare (YIS) and Food Foundation (1985). Growth monitoring as a primary health care activity. Workshop proceedings, 1984. YIS/Ford Foundation, Djarkata.

Fugelsang, A. (1973). *Applied communications in developing countries.* Dag Hammarskjöld Foundation, Uppsala, Sweden.

Genece, E., and Rohde, J. E. (1988). *Ind. J. Ped., 55,* Suppl. 1, S.78. Growth monitoring as an entry point for primary health care.

Ghassemi, H. (Ed.) (1986). Growth of young children, strategies for monitoring and promotion. UNICEF Consultation, 1985. UNICEF, New York.

Ghosh, S. (1988). *Ind. J. Ped., 55,* Suppl. 1, S.67. Growth monitoring—lessons from India.

Gómez, F. Ramos Galvan, R., Frenk, S., Muñoz, J. C., Chaves, R., and Vazquez (1956). *J. Trop. Pediat, 2,* 77. Mortality in second and third degree malnutrition.

Gopalan, C. (1987a). *Bull. Nutr. Found. India, 8,* 37. Growth monitoring: Some basic issues.

Gopalan, C. (1987b). *Bull. Nutr. Found. India, 8,* 37. Choosing "beneficiaries" for funding programmes.

*Gopalan, C., and Chatterjee, M. (1985). Use of growth charts in promoting child nutrition: A review of global experiences. *Nutr. Found. India,* Spec. Publ. Ser. 2.

Gracey, M. (1987). *Wld. Rev. Nutr. Diet, 49:* 160–210. Normal growth and nutrition.

Graitcer, P. L., and Gentry, E. M. (1981). *Lancet, 2,* 297. Measuring children: One reference for all.

Grant, J. (Ed.) (1985). *State of the world's children.* Growth Monitoring, p. 77. UNICEF, New York.

Grant, J. (1987). *State of the world's children.* Going for growth, p. 64. UNICEF, New York.

Grant, J. K., and Stone, T. (1986). *J. Trop. Ped., 32,* 255. Maternal comprehension of a home-based growth chart and its effect on growth.

*Griffiths, M. (1981a). Growth monitoring. American Public Health Association, Washington, D.C.

Griffiths, M. (1981b). Philippine growth table. From USAID Mission Philippines.

Griffiths, M. (1987). *Mothers and Children.* 6, 7. The Bubble Chart.

Griffiths, M. (1988). *Ind. J. Ped., 55,* Suppl. 1, S.59. Growth monitoring—making it a tool for education.

Griffiths, M., and Berg, A. (1989). *Food Nutr. Bull., 10,* 71. The bubble chart: An update on its development.

Guea, E. G., and Lincoln, Y. S. (1981). *Effective evaluation.* Jossey Bass, San Francisco.

*Guilbert, J. J. (1982). *Educational handbook for health personnel* (sixth edition). WHO, Geneva.

Gwatkin, D., Wilcox, J., and Wray, J. (1980). Can health and nutrition interventions make a difference. Monograph res: 13. Overseas Development Council, Washington, D.C.

Hamill, P. V. V., et al. (1979). *Amer. J. Clin. Nutr., 32:* 609–629. National Center for Health Statistics Percentiles.

Hendrata, L. (1988). Growth monitoring and promotion. Guidelines for programming. UNICEF, New York.

Hendrata, L., and Johnson, M. (1978). Manual for community-based under-fives weighing program, Indonesia. Yayasan Indonesia Sejehtera, Jakarta, Indonesia.

Hendrata, L., and Rohde, J. (1988). *Ind. J. Ped.* (Suppl.), *55,* S.9. Ten pitfalls of growth monitoring and promotion.

Hewes, S. (1986). Proposed evaluation study of a growth monitoring program in the Well Child Clinic. Department of Pediatrics, Roosevelt Hospital, Guatemala City, Guatemala.

Jelliffe, D. B. (1956). *J. Ped., 49,* 661. Cultural variation and the practical pediatrician.

Jelliffe, D. B. (1968). Infant nutrition in the subtropics and tropics (second edition). WHO, Geneva.

Jelliffe, D. B. (1986). *Med. J. Malaysia, 41:* 77. Adequacy of lactation: Dysreflexia vs. maternal nutrition.

Jelliffe, D. B., and Jelliffe, E. F. P. (1989c). *Community nutritional assessment.* Oxford University Press, Oxford.

Jelliffe, D. B., and Jelliffe, E. F. P. (1990a). *J. Trop. Ped.* in press. Problems with plotting weight: Newer innovations and a suggested "weight plotter" card.

Jelliffe, D. B., and Jelliffe, E. F. P. (1990b). *J. Trop. Ped.* in press. Colour-coded growth maintenance arm tape for growth monitoring.

Jelliffe, E. F. P. (1968). *Cajanus, 1,* 33. Why do we bother to weigh children?

Jelliffe, E. F. P., and Jelliffe, D. B. (1969). *J. Trop. Ped., 15,* 179. The arm circumference as a public health index of malnutrition.

Jelliffe, E. F. P., and Jelliffe, D. B. (1987). *J. Trop. Ped., 33,* 290. Editorial. Algorithms, growth monitoring and nutritional intervention.

Kigondu, J. G. (1986). How to use the child health card: A guide for health workers in Kenya. Nutrition Division, Ministry of Health, Nairobi, Kenya.

Kittle, B. (1985). *Salubritas, 8,* 4. Designing a growth chart to meet the needs of the community.

Krischer, J. (1980). *Operations Res., 28,* 97. An annotated bibliography of decision analysis applications to health care.

Lakhani, A. D., Avery, A., Gordon, A., and Tait, N. (1984). *Arch. Dis. Childh., 59,* 1096. Evaluation of a home-based health record booklet.

Lancet (1985). *ii,* 1337–8. Editorial: Growth monitoring: intermediate technology or expensive luxury?

Lankester, T. E. (1988). *Trop. Doctor, 18,* 91. Health Shepherding. A system to find and care for the needy minority.

Lovel, H., De Graaf, J., and Gordon G. (1984). *Assignment Children, 65,* 275. How mothers measure growth.

Manoff, R. (1985). *Social marketing: New imperative for public health.* Praeger Press, New York.

Margo, G. (1976). *Amer. J. Ch. Nutr., 29,* 835. Assessing malnutrition with the mid-arm circumference.

Marsden, P. D. (1964). *Trans. Roy. Soc. Trop. Med. Hyg., 58,* 455. The Sukuta Project.

McGuire, J. S. and Austin, J. E. (1987). Beyond survival: children's growth for national development. UNICEF, New York.

McLaren, D. S. (1987). *Wld. Rev. Nutr. Diet., 49,* 87–120. A fresh look at some perinatal growth and nutritional standards.

McMahon, R., Barton, E., and Piot, M. (1980). On being in charge: A guide for middle-level management in primary health care. WHO, Geneva.

Morley, D. C. (1968). *Trop. Geogr. Med., 20,* 101. Health and weight chart for use in developing countries.

Morley, D. C. (1977). *Arch. Dis. Childh., 52,* 395. Growth charts—"curative" or "preventive."

Morley, D. C., and Woodland, M. (1979). *See how they grow.* Macmillan, London.

Morley, D. C. (1986) *Bull. Internat. Ped. Assoc., 383.* Optimal growth and monitoring.

Morrow, H. (1985). Report on post-workshop projects: Mobilizing nursing leadership for primary health care. International Council of Nurses, Geneva.

Moteetee, M. M. (1989) Personal communication.

Nabarro, D., and Chinnock, P. (1988) *Soc. Sci. Med., 26,* 941. Growth monitoring—inappropriate promotion of an appropriate technology.

Program for Appropriate Technology in Health (PATH) (1983). *Health Technology Directions, 3,* 1. Assessing nutritional status: Practical measures for primary health care.

Program for Appropriate Technology in Health (PATH) (1987). *Health Technology Directions, 7,* 1. Traditional media.

Roche, A. F., and Hines, J. H. (1980). *Amer. J. Clin. Nutr., 33,* 8041. Incremental growth charts.

*Rohde, J. E. (Ed.) (1988). *Ind. J. Ped. 55,* Suppl. 1, S.1-S.123. Symposium: Growth monitoring and promotion: An international perspective.

Rohde, J. E., Ismail, D., and Sutrisno, R. (1978). *J. Trop. Ped., 51,* 295. Mothers as weight-watchers.

Rohde, J. E., Ismail, D., Sadjimin, T., Suyadi, A., and Tugerin (1979). *J. Trop. Ped., 52,* 83. Training course for village nutrition programs.

Rohde, J. E., and Northrup, R. S. (1985). *Ind. J. Ped., 55,* Suppl. 1, S.110. Feeding, feedback and sustenance of primary health care.

Scrimshaw, S., and Hurtado, E. (1987). *Rapid assessment procedures for nutrition and primary health care.* Anthropological approaches to programme improvement. United Nations University and UCLA Latin American Center, Los Angeles.

Segall, M. (1979). *Lancet, i,* 1352. Growth charts for developing countries.

Sempé, M., and Masse, N. (1965). Methodes de measures et resultats. In Proc. XX Congres de l'Association des Pediatres de Langue Francaise, Nancy. International Children's Centre, Paris.

Sénécal, J., and Roussey, M. (1976). *Concours medical, 98,* 1734. Comment remplir le carnet de santé.

Shakir, A., and Morley, D. (1974). *Lancet, i,* 758. Measuring malnutrition.

*Shorr, I. J. (1985). How to weigh and measure children. National household capability programme. United Nations Department of Technical Cooperation for Development and Statistics, New York.

Shorr, I. J. (1989). A critique of four hanging spring scales suitable for field use. PVO (Private Voluntary Organizations) Child Survival Workshop, Lake Junaluska, N.C.

Shu-fang, L., and Wei-zhi, D. (1989). *Chinese Med. J., 102,* 233. A growth velocity standard for Chinese children in Hong Kong.

Sinha, D. (1987). Personal communication. CFNI, Jamaica.

Sinha, D. (1986). A system for monitoring nutritional status and actions to improve children's health. A field guide for health workers in the Caribbean. CFNI/PAHO, Kingston, Jamaica.

Srilatha, V. L. (1986). *Bull. Nutr. Found. India, 7,* 6. Use of growth charts for promoting child nutrition.

Srinivasan, L. (1982). Bridging the gap: A participatory approach to health and nutrition. Save the Children, USA.

Steveny, J. (1982). *Trop. Doctor, 12,* 133. Standardized interpretation of under-5 weight curves.

Storms, D. M. (1979). Training and use of auxiliary health workers: Lessons from developing countries. APHA, International Health Programs Monograph Series No. 3.

Sukmanah, Titi. (1987). Growth monitoring as individual and community nutrition education: The Indonesian experience. WHO/IUNS Workshop, CFNI, Jamaica.

Taymor, C. E. (1988). *Ind. J. Ped., 55,* Suppl. 1, S.16. Child growth as a community surveillance indicator.

Teller, C., Yee, V., and More, J. D. (1985). Growth monitoring as a useful primary health care management tool. Proc. Meeting Council for Internat. Hlth., Washington, D.C.

Teller, C., Yee, V., and Mora, J. D. (1987). *Child Survival Action News, 7.* Growth Monitoring: A child's "Road to Health" report card.

Thurm, A. T. (1988). Qualitative research for animated health messages project. UNICEF, New York.

Tremlitt, G., Lovel, H., and Morley, D. C. (1983). *Assignment Children.* No: 61/62. Guidelines for the design of national weight-for-ages growth charts.

Tulchinsky, T. H., Acker, C., El Malki, K., Socolar, R. S., and Reshef, A. (1985). *Bull. Wld. Hlth. Org., 63,* 1137. Use of growth chart as a simple epidemiological monitoring system of nutritional status of children.

UNICEF (1985). How to use the child health card. A guide for health workers in Swaziland. Ministry of Health, Mbabane, Swaziland.

U.S. Agency for International Development (1972). *Evaluation handbook* (second edition). AID Office and Program Evaluation, Washington, D.C.

U.S. Agency for International Development (1988). Growth monitoring and nutrition education. Office of Nutrition, USAID, Washington, D.C.

Vella, J. K. (1982). *Learning to listen.* Center for International Education, University of Massachusetts.

Waterlow, J. C., Ashworth, A., and Griffiths, M. (1980). *Lancet, ii,* 1176. Faltering in growth in less-developed countries.

Werner, D., and Bower, B. (1982). *Helping health workers to learn.* Hesperian Foundation, Palo Alto, Calif.

Wilkinson, K. N. (1982). *Trans. Roy. Soc. Trop. Med. Hyg., 76,* 77. A damping system for under fives weighing scales.

Williams, C. D., Baumslag, N., and Jelliffe, D. B. (1986). *Mother and child health: Delivering the services* (second edition). Oxford University Press, Oxford.

Wit, J. M., Davies, C., and Molthof, J. (1984). *Trop. Doctor, 14,* 36. Introduction of a home- and clinic-based growth chart in Dominica.

*World Federation of Public Health Associations (1983a). *Training community health workers.* UNICEF, New York.

World Federation of Public Health Associations (1983b). Synopses of community health workers (CHW) trained in selected projects. UNICEF, New York.

World Health Organization (1978a). Alma-Ata 1978. Primary health care. WHO, Geneva.

*World Health Organization (1978b). A growth chart for international use in maternal and child care: Guidelines for primary health care personnel. WHO, Geneva.

World Health Organization (1983a). *Measuring change in nutritional status.* Guidelines for assessing the nutritional impact of supplementary feeding programmes for vulnerable groups. WHO, Geneva.

World Health Organization (1983b). Training in recording the child's growth. Document EPI/PHW/83/TM.1/Rev. 2.

World Health Organization (1985a). A guide to curriculum review for basic nursing education: Orientation of primary health care and community health. WHO, Geneva.

World Health Organization (1985b). Report of the consultative group on the organization of health systems based on primary health care. Doc. SHS/86.2. WHO, Geneva.

*World Health Organization (1986a). The growth chart. A tool for use in infant and child care. WHO, Geneva.

World Health Organization (1986b). Guidelines for training community health workers in nutrition (second edition). WHO, Geneva.

World Health Organization (1987). The community health care worker. WHO, Geneva.

World Health Organization (1989). Growth performance: Decision-making skills for selecting appropriate actions (in prep). WHO, Geneva.

Wray, J. (1986). Report of discussions of certain aspects of growth monitoring from a small workshop held at UNICEF, New York, April 1986.

Yost, D. A., and Pust, R. E. (1987). *J. Trop. Ped.*, *34*, 15. Arm circumference as an index of protein-energy malnutrition in six-to-eleven-month-old rural Tanzanian children.

Zeitlin, M. (1986). *J. Trop. Ped.*, *22*, 190. Comparison of malnourished children selected by weight-for-age, mid-upper arm circumference and maximum thigh circumference.

Zeitlin, M. Beiser, A., and Weld, L. (1987). Policy implications of a project to investigate misclassification errors in growth monitoring. Unpublished manuscript.

Zeitlin, M. F., Pyle, D. F., Austin, J. E., Sempore, G., and Gouba, E. (1982). *J. Trop. Ped.*, *28*, 62. Circumference growth charts for community level workers with little or no formal schooling.

Zerfas, A. J. (1975). *Amer. J. Clin. Nutr.*, *28*, 782. The insertion tape.

Zerfas, A. J. (1985). Checking continuous measures. Manual for examiners, School of Public Health, University of California, Los Angeless.

Zerfas, A. J. (1986). Decisions for health interventions. A manual for trainers and supervisors. LTS/International Nutrition Unit, Rockville, Md.

Index